Missouri and Arkansas Campground Locator Map

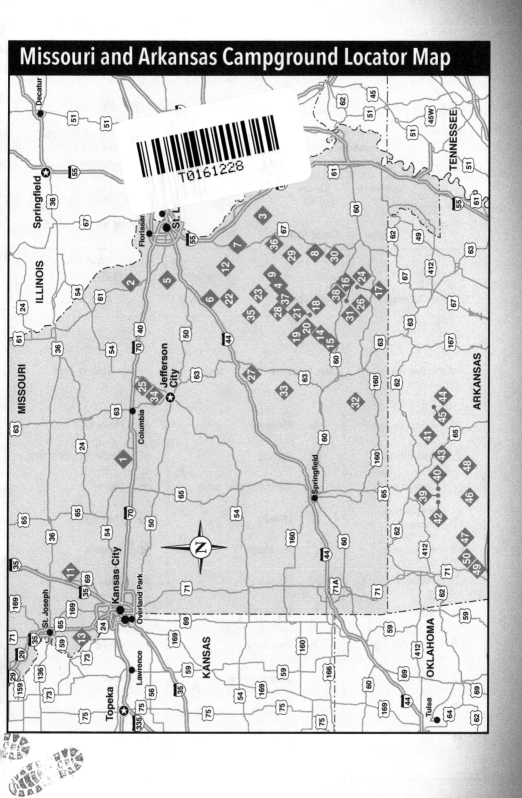

Missouri & The Ozarks Campground Map Legend

 North indicator

Off-map or pinpoint-indication arrow

Campground name and location

Individual tents, walk-in sites, cottages, cabins, and lean-to within campground area

Group site

Jefferson City ✪ **Capital**

Kansas City ○ **City or town**

NATIONAL FOREST STATE PARK
Public lands

Main Trail
Hiking trails

Steps

(55) **Interstate highways**

(67) **US highways**

(34)-(CC)-(143) **State roads**

Quail Rd.
CR 425 FS 2266
Other roads

Dirt/gravel roads

Area boundary

Creek
River or stream

Lake
Lake or pond

⋈ Bridge or tunnel	Playground	Picnic area
Amphitheater	P Parking	Sheltered picnic area
Water access	Marina or boat ramp	Lodge
Wheelchair accessible	Laundry	Fishing area
Restroom	Telephone	Showers
Pit toilet	Horse trail	Dump station
Store	$ Pay station	Peak
Trash disposal	Swimming	Spring
Overlook	Ranger station	Gate
Beach	Firewood	Water entry point
Dining	Fire tower	Dam

OVERVIEW MAP KEY

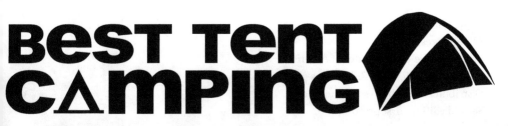

BEST TENT CAMPING

MISSOURI
& THE OZARKS

YOUR CAR-CAMPING GUIDE TO SCENIC BEAUTY, THE SOUNDS OF NATURE, AND AN ESCAPE FROM CIVILIZATION

2nd Edition

STEVE HENRY

MENASHA RIDGE PRESS
Your Guide to the Outdoors Since 1982

Best Tent Camping: Missouri & the Ozarks

Copyright © 2014 by Steve Henry
All rights reserved
Printed in the United States of America
Published by Menasha Ridge Press
Distributed by Publishers Group West
Second edition, first printing

Library of Congress Cataloging-in-Publication Data

Henry, Steve.
  The best in tent camping. Missouri and the Ozarks : your car-camping guide to scenic beauty, the sounds of nature, and an escape from civilization / Steve Henry.
     pages cm
  ISBN 978-0-89732-644-5 (pbk.) — ISBN 0-89732-644-X
  ISBN 978-1-63404-191-1 (hardcover) — ISBN 978-0-89732-676-6 (ebook)
  1. Camp sites, facilities, etc.—Ozark Mountains—Guidebooks. 2. Camping—Ozark Mountains—Guidebooks. 3. Ozark Mountains--Guidebooks. 4. Camp sites, facilities, etc.—Missouri—Guidebooks. 5. Camping—Missouri—Guidebooks. 6. Missouri—Guidebooks. I. Title.
  GV199.42.O96H45 2013
  917.67'1--dc23
                              2013041714

Cover design by Scott McGrew
Text design by Annie Long
Cover photo by © Aurora Photos/Alamy
Cartography by Steve Jones
Indexing by Rich Carlson
Author photo by Glenn Meyer

🏵 **MENASHA RIDGE PRESS**
An imprint of AdventureKEEN
2204 First Avenue South, Suite 102
Birmingham, Alabama 35233
menasharidge.com

CONTENTS

● ●

AUTHOR'S TOP CAMPGROUNDS

:: BEST FOR SCENIC BEAUTY AND PHOTOGRAPHY

:: BEST FOR SWIMMING

ACKNOWLEDGMENTS

● ●

Thanks, of course, to all the usual suspects—my family and friends, who gave me constant encouragement, and the folks at Menasha, who waited patiently as I missed one deadline and pushed against another, and then turned this mountain of information into an attractive and organized guidebook. Thanks also to all of you who enjoy the outdoors, and by doing so have made this book a success over the years. Special thanks to Chuck, my boss and brother, who lets live where I work, thus freeing up the time and money I need for travel, research, and writing, and to my good friends Brian, Larry, and Lucy, who graciously let me stay at their homes when I'm doing book research in their area. And a disbelieving thanks to the two strangers who complimented my banjo playing that night at Paddy Creek Campground—you must have known it was my birthday, and just wanted to make me feel good.

These are times of shrinking budgets, sequesters, shutdowns, and political battles over government spending. While researching this book, my thoughts often went to the park, conservation department, and forest service employees who work hard in the face of dwindling resources to keep our campgrounds, trails, and other outdoor treasures open and available for our enjoyment. Their dedication reminded me of the 1930s Civilian Conservation Corps, young men whose superb craftsmanship and long-abandoned camps can be found in many campgrounds described in this book, and evoked thoughts of John McCutcheon's ode to the CCC, "Boys In Green." So above all, many thanks to the boys, and the gals too, in green, who keep our country's natural wonders open and accessible to all.

In Nineteen Hundred and Thirty Three
Off in Washington, DC
Roosevelt created the CCC
Like nothing we'd ever seen

He called on fellers across the land
To join together, lend a hand
To learn a skill, to take a stand
We were the boys in green

Hurrah for the love of the country
Hurrah for the patriot's dream
With their brains and their backs, with a pick and an axe
Hurrah for the boys in green

©2003 by John McCutcheon/Appalsongs (ASCAP)
Inspired in part by a conversation with O'Neal Springer, Dallas, TX, October 2003

PREFACE

● ●

I had a blast cruising scenic and winding Ozark highways while researching these beautiful campgrounds. My only regret was not having time to spend several days in each one. Now that this edition is finished, I can do what I hope is in the cards for you—spend several seasons checking out these wonderful hideaways in the Ozark Mountains. I've hiked or biked most trails mentioned in these chapters and paddled more than a few of the rivers. On my wanderings I've meandered along forested mountainsides, gazed awestruck from 500-foot bluffs, picnicked in rocky glades, explored spectacular caves, stared deep into aquamarine springs, and napped in meadows of wildflowers.

From these campgrounds you can also experience those Missouri and Arkansas backcountry pleasures. Thousands of miles of streams await your fishing pole and canoe and paddle. These cool, spring-fed rivers and creeks are the perfect antidote to the heat and humidity of summer, and several of the sparkling-clear springs are among the largest in the world. All are accessible by car, canoe, or a short hike. When the weather cools, it's time to get out of the river and explore the rugged countryside on hundreds of miles of hiking and mountain biking trails.

Don't stop your camping exploration with these 50 campgrounds—many more scenic hideaways await you in the Ozarks. Nor should you let the off-season weather limit your camping season. You'll see better views from overlooks when the leaves are off the trees. Cooler temperatures also mean no bugs or crowded campgrounds. Winter skies offer incredible stargazing, and in December and January the remote mountains are perfect for enjoying two of the heavens' biggest meteor showers. I'll never forget winter camping next to a southwest Missouri creek, where ice columns 3 feet thick towered 100 feet over the streambed from an overlooking bluff. During winter, I'm thankful to live in the Midwest instead of the Rockies. When campgrounds and trails in those spectacular Western mountains are choked with snow, I can still wander the Ozark hills.

Don't take my word for it—pick up this book and a couple of trail guides, round up some maps, toss your camping gear into the car, and head for the hills to see for yourself. Hope to see you out there!

—Steve Henry

INTRODUCTION

● ●

How to Use This Guidebook

The publishers of Menasha Ridge Press welcome you to *Best Tent Camping: Missouri and the Ozarks*. Whether you're new to this activity or you've been sleeping in your portable outdoor shelter over decades of outdoor adventures, please review the following information. It explains how we have worked with the author to organize this book and how you can make the best use of it.

Some passages in this introduction are applicable to all of the books in the Best Tent Camping guidebook series. Where this isn't the case, such as in the descriptions of weather, wildlife, and plants, the author has provided information specific to your area.

:: THE RATINGS & RATING CATEGORIES

As with all of the books in the publisher's Best Tent Camping series, this guidebook's author personally experienced dozens of campgrounds and campsites to select the top 50 locations in this region. Within that universe of 50 sites, the author then ranked each one in the six categories described below. Each campground in this guidebook is superlative in its own way. For example, a site may be rated only one star in one category but perhaps five stars in another category. This rating system allows you to choose your destination based on the attributes that are most important to you. Though these ratings are subjective, they're still excellent guidelines for finding the perfect camping experience for you and your companions. Below and following we describe the criteria for each of the attributes in our five-star rating system:

★ ★ ★ ★ ★   The site is **ideal** in that category.
★ ★ ★ ★   The site is **exemplary** in that category.
★ ★ ★   The site is **very good** in that category.
★ ★   The site is **above average** in that category.
★   The site is **acceptable** in that category.

Beauty

All 50 campgrounds in this guide are wonderful places. In the Ozarks, the most beautiful campgrounds overlook one of the scenic rivers meandering through the forested hills, often with bluffs towering near the campsites. Others are on mountaintops. Even those with fewer than five stars are comfortable hideaways that you'll hate to leave on hiking, canoeing, biking, or other explorations in the surrounding Ozark Mountains.

Privacy

I'm really particular on this feature. For an outdoor misanthrope like me, few campgrounds have sites far enough apart. Campgrounds with good spacing and brushy growth between the sites offer the best seclusion, and many of the hideaways in this guide fill that bill. Some do not, but I included them because they were in beautiful settings or had lots of nearby outdoor activities from which to choose. In general, you'll find that state and national parks offer the least privacy, and national forests offer the most.

Spaciousness

Some folks like open space around their campsite. Even if they have the most private site on the planet, they still feel crowded if their car, table, and tent are jammed too closely together. Others camp with friends and thus need room for two or three tents on their site. Camping spots rated high in this category are usually level sites with grassy open spaces surrounding them, often with a nice view of the adjacent countryside.

Quiet

This is another big one for me. Most of the campgrounds included here are far from roads, towns, railroads, and the like, so they're very peaceful. The wild card is you and your neighbors. In the hushed settings where you'll find these campgrounds, one loud group can ruin things for everyone. Avoid three-day summer weekends and nearby festivals and you'll almost always enjoy peace and quiet in these Ozark enclaves.

Security

Unless there's a heavy ranger or host presence, you need to watch your stuff no matter where you camp. Consequently, few campgrounds get a five-star rating. On the other hand, just one received fewer than four stars, and that was only because signs warning campers to lock their valuables were posted in the campground. Ozark campgrounds are usually as safe as they are beautiful, especially if you keep your camp buttoned up and neat while you are away enjoying the outdoors. And don't forget security from our four-legged and feathered friends too. Keep a clean camp and you won't come home to a shambles made by marauding raccoons, squirrels, blue jays, or bears.

Cleanliness

Almost every campground in this guide rates five stars. Only a few do not, and they are usually the most remote and unvisited sites. These out-of-the-way campgrounds are very beautiful but just don't get as much attention from either campers or maintenance crews as their well-manicured brethren. They are often my favorites for that very reason. Overall, you'll be impressed with the clean and attractive appearance of these Ozark homes-away-from-home.

:: THE OVERVIEW MAP, MAP KEY, AND LEGEND

Use the overview map on the inside front cover to assess the exact location of each campground. The campground's number appears not only on the overview map but also on the map key facing the overview map, in the table of contents, and on the profile's first page. This book is organized by agency, as indicated in the table of contents.

A map legend that details the symbols found on the campground-layout maps appears on the inside back cover.

:: CAMPGROUND-LAYOUT MAPS

Each profile includes a detailed map of campground sites, internal roads, facilities, and other key items.

:: GPS CAMPGROUND-ENTRANCE COORDINATES

Readers can easily access all campgrounds in this book by using the directions given and the overview map, which shows at least one major road leading into the area. But for those who enjoy using GPS technology to navigate, the book includes coordinates for each campground's entrance in latitude and longitude, expressed in degrees and decimal minutes. To convert GPS coordinates from degrees, minutes, and seconds to the above degrees–decimal minutes format, the seconds are divided by 60. For more on GPS technology, visit **usgs.gov.**

A note of caution: Actual GPS devices will easily guide you to any of these campgrounds, but users of smartphone mapping apps will find that cell phone service is often unavailable in the hills and hollows where many of these hideaways are located.

:: THE CAMPGROUND PROFILE

Each profile contains a concise but informative narrative of the campground and individual sites. Not only is the property described, but also readers can get a general idea of the recreational opportunities available—what's in the area and perhaps suggestions for touristy activities. This descriptive text is enhanced with three helpful sidebars: Ratings, Key Information, and Getting There (accurate driving directions that lead you to the campground from the nearest major roadway, along with GPS coordinates).

About This Book

Welcome to the rugged hills and hollows of the Ozarks, where you'll find some of the prettiest campgrounds in America. This is a land of clear rivers, tall bluffs, deep forests, and aquamarine springs. Hundreds of miles of trails and thousands of miles of rivers lace the countryside around these scenic forest camps, waiting for you to explore on hiking, biking, or paddling adventures.

Haunting reminders of the past will pique your interest in these Ozark hideaways. Many of the campgrounds were built by the Civilian Conservation Corps (CCC) in the 1930s, and they showcase the unique native stone and wood architecture for which CCC projects are famous. Several of the campgrounds are actual sites of old CCC camps, where you can wander past crumbling foundations and chimneys from the long-gone work camps whose legacies we still enjoy 70 years later.

Other common remnants of old times in the Ozarks are the numerous mill sites scattered throughout the hills. It seems that every campground in the Ozarks once had a mill operating nearby. Nearly every stream or spring large enough to roll a waterwheel once powered a mill to grind corn, saw logs, gin cotton, or card wool for the farmers working their hardscrabble Ozark lands. Some of these mills are gone without a trace. At others you can find remnants of the dams and raceways but little else. Several are still standing, dilapidated ghosts, and a few, such as Alley Mill and Dillard Mill, are restored historic structures.

:: MISSOURI STATE PARKS

Missouri has beautiful state parks that are very worthy of a visit. Unfortunately, campsites in these state-park campgrounds are often packed a little too tightly together and are popular on summer weekends, and the parks themselves are sometimes overdeveloped. They typically offer less privacy than their national forest and national river counterparts and attract more RV campers. Still, I included 12 state-park campgrounds. These parks are either too scenic or interesting to be left out, or their campgrounds are more laid-back than most. They're nice places to be even during the busy summer months, but off-season camping in Missouri's state parks is especially easygoing and delightful. One especially wonderful feature of Missouri's state park system is its website. Each park has its own Web page with tons of information on the park, including a link to up-to-date temperature and weather forecasts, and most pages include a short video describing the park's attractions. Go to the park Web page's campground map and click on the site you're considering, and up pops a window with specifications on that site such as shade, degree of slope, size of the parking pad, and more—including a button to click for a photo of the site.

:: U.S. FOREST SERVICE

Site for site, the best tent camping in this book is found within the Mark Twain and Ozark National Forests. While the state and national parks sport more amenities, the forest service campgrounds are usually quieter, offer more private sites, and generally have the more rustic, way-out-there feel that's so suitable for tent camping. Two-thirds of them have no electric sites, many have only pit toilets, and a few don't even have water, thus keeping the RV crowd out of your hair. These campgrounds are often located near wonderful canoeing streams and superb hiking and mountain biking trails, and a few of them don't even charge a fee. For the most solitude, choose one of the six forest camps at the end of long drives on gravel roads, like my two favorites—Paddy Creek in Missouri and Richland Creek in Arkansas.

:: NATIONAL PARK SERVICE

Campgrounds in Arkansas's Buffalo National River and Missouri's Ozark National Scenic Riverways are administered by the National Park Service. The 2013 budget sequester forced closure of several campgrounds and curtailed seasons and services in some others. These changes are indefinite, and the park service hopes to reinstate services and reopen closed campgrounds once the budget problems are sorted out. Things were still in a state of flux as this guide went to press, with some year-round campgrounds being considered for shortened seasons. Check the park's website before planning an off-season camping trip—hopefully you'll find that not only is your chosen campground open, but access has been restored to the others too.

:: ELECTRICITY'S INCURSION INTO OZARK CAMPGROUNDS

It has been well over 200 years since Ben Franklin made his probably mythical kite-flying breakthrough, and electricity is finally finding its way into more and more campgrounds in the Ozarks. I'm thankful that it has taken this long, but electrified campsites are unfortunately becoming more widespread in Missouri and Arkansas with each passing year—dramatically so since the previous edition of this guide in 2005. It has shown up in many campgrounds where it was nonexistent then, and some of the state park camps have been almost completely electrified. Officials say they're only giving people what they want, and it's probably true. In most campgrounds where it's offered, the electric sites usually have a higher occupancy rate than the more basic ones. Perhaps in our age of laptops, smartphones, tablets, video games, and TV, this evolution was inevitable. On a positive note, it seems to be drawing more families to the outdoors, and maybe the kids will grow up to be hikers, bicyclists, and canoeists who end up preferring tents to RVs. Happily, most campgrounds with electricity still offer basic loops for tent campers in a separate area, but expect to sometimes share your campground with the RV crowd.

:: WEATHER

All seasons are wonderful for camping in the Ozarks. Though summer is often hot and humid, the rivers, swimming holes, and lakes at most campgrounds keep campers comfortable in even the worst heat wave. Spring is a beautiful time to be outdoors in the Ozarks—wildflowers are everywhere, dogwood and redwood blooms brighten the gray forest, turkeys gobble in the early morning, and spring peepers serenade you from the lakes and streams near camp. Fall is nearly everyone's favorite. Cold, frosty mornings chip away at the lassitude left from summer's heat. In fall's crisp air you begin breathing easily and deeply for the first time in months, and your body wakes up ready to hit the trails. Pleasing hues of orange, red, yellow, and caramel decorate the forest as the trees prepare to shed their summer foliage. Next to fall, I really enjoy winter camping. The humidity, heat, bugs, and crowds are gone; the streams are shallow and easier to cross; and the bare trees open up scenic views obscured by lush foliage during the warmer months.

:: FIRST-AID KIT

A useful first-aid kit may contain more items than you might think necessary. These are just the basics. Prepackaged kits in waterproof bags (Atwater Carey and Adventure Medical make them) are available. As a preventive measure, take along sunscreen and insect repellent. Even though quite a few items are listed here, they pack down into a small space:

- Ace bandages or Spenco joint wraps
- Adhesive bandages, such as Band-Aids
- Antibiotic ointment (*Neosporin or the generic equivalent*)
- Antiseptic or disinfectant, such as Betadine or hydrogen peroxide
- Aspirin, acetaminophen, or ibuprofen
- Benadryl or the generic equivalent, diphenhydramine (*in case of allergic reactions*)
- Butterfly-closure bandages

(continued on next page)

(First-Aid Kit continued)

- Comb and tweezers (*for removing ticks from your skin*)
- Dark chocolate (*won't cure anything, but it'll sure make you feel better*)
- Epinephrine in a prefilled syringe (*for severe allergic reactions to such things as bee stings*)
- Gauze (*one roll and six 4- by 4-inch compress pads*)
- LED flashlight or headlamp
- Matches or lighter
- Moist towelettes
- Moleskin/Spenco 2nd Skin
- Pocketknife or multipurpose tool
- Waterproof first-aid tape
- Whistle (*it's more effective in signaling rescuers than your voice*)

:: ANIMAL AND PLANT HAZARDS

Bears

Ursus Americanus, the American black bear, was reintroduced into Arkansas around 1960. Though not common, they're out there, especially in the more remote regions of Arkansas's Boston Mountains and Buffalo River area, and an occasional bruin finds its way into southern Missouri. Normal precautions for keeping nuisance animals such as raccoons out of your food supply are usually all that's necessary when camping in the Ozarks. Check campground bulletin boards when you pull into camp—a notice, along with additional precautions you should take, will be posted if recent bear activity has occurred in the camp or its surrounding area.

Emerald Ash Borer

This exotic insect, a native of Asia, has already killed millions of ash trees in the northern United States. It has been detected in several Missouri counties and is threatening to move into Arkansas. Its spread is aided by transportation of wood around the state. To combat its spread, burn only firewood gathered or purchased near your campsite, as directed under the "Restrictions" category in the Key Information box on nearly every campground profile. Burn all your firewood before you break camp, and don't leave any for other campers.

Poison Ivy

This little three-leaf villain is just as common in the Ozarks as the tick, but easier to avoid because it stays in one place rather than coming after you. Watch for its three-leaf configuration, both in ground cover and vines on trees near your campsite. Within 14 hours of exposure you'll have blisters and a terrible itch in the affected area. Wash and dry the area thoroughly with alcohol, soap, and water as soon as possible after exposure. Wearing long pants and sleeves will help protect you, but be careful—touching your clothing or even pets or camping gear that have contacted poison ivy may spread the plant's rash-producing oil onto your skin. If you're sensitive to the ivy's effects, bring along one of the various over-the-counter products that alleviate poison ivy's irritating symptoms.

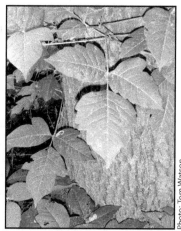

Photo: Tom Watson

Snakes

Venomous snakes aren't a huge problem in the Ozarks, but they're out there. Copperheads are the most common. Rattlesnakes, while rare, are occasionally sighted in the Ozarks. You may spot cottonmouth water moccasins in streams, lakes, and even in pools along trails. Unless they're torpid from cold weather, snakes will see you or sense your footfalls before you reach them and move away.

Ticks

If ticks bother you, you can't camp in the Ozarks. They're ubiquitous, just part of the deal when enjoying the outdoors in Missouri and Arkansas. You can contract Lyme disease and Rocky Mountain spotted fever from these annoying little critters, but it rarely happens, especially if you're vigilant and remove them soon after they find you. Wearing light-colored clothing makes them easier to spot, and an insect repellent with DEET helps keep them away. Ticks prefer places where they're held tightly against your skin, such as elastic on socks and underwear, your underarms, waistband, and back of the knee. Tweezers are ideal for removing ticks that have already attached—just grab it as close to the skin surface as possible and firmly pull it loose without crushing it. Expect a bit of redness and itching for a few days around the bite site.

:: CAMPING ETIQUETTE

Here are a few tips on how to create good vibes with fellow campers and wildlife you encounter:

- **Be a good neighbor**. Keep the peace—don't play music or party loudly, even if it's not quiet hours. Get to camp before everyone goes to bed. If you must arrive late, set up quietly with a minimum of talk and bright lights shining all over the place. Avoid loud and boisterous banter that disturbs your neighbors, keep your dog leashed and quiet, and don't hike through someone else's site just to save yourself a few steps. In other words, camp by the Golden Rule.

- **Leave only footprints.** Deposit garbage in the Dumpster, not around your campsite or in the fire ring. Don't cut trees in and around your campsite, or hammer nails into them for hanging your gear. Wipe off your table, clean up bits of trash as you depart, and leave the place as clean as you'd like to see it the next time you visit.

- **Obtain all authorizations and permits required.** Check in, pay your fee, and occupy your site as directed on the campground's signboard. If you see a site you like better than your own, be sure it's not reserved before you make your move. If in doubt, check with the campground host. At self-serve campgrounds with no host, don't skip out without paying your fee. Such questionable behavior only results in higher fees, more stringent rules, and perhaps the closure of less-frequented campgrounds that offer excellent tent camping.

- **Follow the rules.** Observe rules regarding parking, check-out times, and number of people, tents, or vehicles per site. If you need an exception, just ask. Most hosts and agencies accommodate special requests if at all possible. Pay special attention to guidelines regarding fires—bans may be in effect due to drought, and firewood restrictions are in place to limit the spread of the emerald ash borer. And please don't burn your trash in the fire ring—you'll stink up the whole campground and make about as many friends as I do when I play the banjo in my campsite.

:: TIPS FOR A HAPPY CAMPING TRIP

- **Do some legwork.** During the peak camping season, make reservations at popular campgrounds to ensure you get a campsite. Off-season, make sure your chosen campground is open. Because I'm a winter camper, I wish all campgrounds stayed open year-round. Sadly, some of the most beautiful do not. Seasons stated in each campground profile were current at press time, but beware of changes in seasons, fees, dates of water availability, and campground facilities. Campgrounds are constantly being improved, renovated, and, occasionally, closed. Especially dicey are dates of water availability. At some year-round campgrounds, weather dictates when the water supply is turned on and off. When in doubt, call or check the website for the agency operating the campground. That way you'll never be caught short.

- **Avoid holidays.** I always invoke the three-day weekend rule—Just Say No to Camping on Memorial Day, July Fourth, or Labor Day weekends. At these times campgrounds are almost always full. Avoid weekends when a nearby special event might fill the campground you are considering. I've noted these when possible, but you just never know when you're going to stumble on the Rock-and-Roll Rappers Reunion Party and Campout at your chosen getaway site. But lucky you—if you have this book, you'll always be able to find a nice alternative, won't you? Camp during the week whenever possible and you'll often have one of these Ozark hideaways all to yourself.

- **Delve into local history.** My most enjoyable camping experiences happen when I learn about and explore the countryside around my campground. To me, exploring a landscape without knowing about it is like reading a book in a foreign language–I can admire the pretty pictures, but I can't read the deeper and more fascinating story behind them. The information in this book, extensive as I've tried to make it, barely scratches the surface. Doing some digging on your own really draws you into your environment. Local histories abound nowadays, and their stories make fascinating campground reading. Shooting the breeze with residents in local bars and restaurants is another fun way to pick up bits of local lore.

- **Study nature.** I always carry plant and wildlife guides with me when I camp. These resources truly open up the outdoors to me, helping me understand what flowers, bugs, birds, and other critters I'm seeing when I'm out there camping, hiking, biking, and paddling the Ozarks. Without those guides my travels would be much less interesting and full of unanswered questions about what's growing by the trail, singing in the treetops, or crawling up my leg.

- **Get out and explore.** Reading these chapters, you'll find constant references to routes for mountain biking and hiking and rivers for canoeing and fishing. I've given brief descriptions for many, but you'll need more information to really find your way. The bibliography at the end of this book lists excellent guides that will tell you of the great trails and riverways awaiting you in the Ozarks. A few are out of print but can still easily be found on Amazon or eBay. I also recommend obtaining national forest maps. They're great for leading you on otherwise confusing scenic drives and finding your way on backcountry mountain bike routes. The Trails Illustrated maps of the Buffalo National River and the Ozark National Scenic Riverways are wonderful resources for navigating those Ozark gems. Before heading outdoors, contact or check websites for the forest service, state parks, and national river offices. They have free maps of many of the trails mentioned in this guide and often sell the trail guides listed in the bibliography. Armed with some of these guides, you can explore the countryside and stay on the right path.

May your campsite always be peaceful, shady, spacious, level, and free of mosquitoes. Have fun out there!

State and County Parks

1

Arrow Rock
State Historic Site

Arrow Rock State Historic Site offers a peek into central Missouri's early 19th-century history.

Unlike the landscapes surrounding most campgrounds in this book, Arrow Rock isn't a natural scenic wonder. Its campground is still a peaceful hideaway, but the area's draw is its history. The town's name is derived from the nearby bluffs visible for miles on the Missouri River, which were noted on a 1732 French explorers map as Pierre a Flèche, or "rock of arrows."

Travelers on the Santa Fe Trail, who replenished their water supply at the spring behind the Old Tavern, used a ferry built near Arrow Rock in 1815. Initially founded under the name New Philadelphia, Arrow Rock was home to several notable Americans, including Dr. John Sappington, who discovered quinine as an effective malaria treatment, and artist George Caleb Bingham, who used town scenes in several of his paintings. By the mid-1800s Arrow Rock's population was around 1,000, but the combined effects of the Civil War, declining steamboat traffic, and the bypassing of Arrow Rock by the railroad industry

caused the town to dwindle. Though fewer than 100 souls now inhabit Arrow Rock, its past still lives through its old buildings, antiques shops, and historic sites.

Arrow Rock's campground is just south of town, and all sites are an easy walk from Arrow Rock's Main Street. The loop containing sites 1–12 is closest to the town, and all its sites are basic, nonelectric camping spots in a tight circle under a grove of trees. Sites 1 (an accessible site) and 2 are the most level and spacious campsites in the loop, but they're the least shaded. Site 3 has better shade but does not really have a good spot for your tent. Sites 4, 5, and 6 have plenty of grassy space around them and decent shade, but they're somewhat tightly spaced and are on gently sloping terrain. Sites 7, 8, 11, and 12 don't have level tent spots, but would be good campsites for camper vans or pop-ups. Sites 9 and 10 are close together, but they do have enough level grassy space for tents.

The sites in the first loop are good for avoiding RVs, but if you don't mind being with the RV crowd, you'll find flatter and more spacious tent sites in the south part of the campground. It's about a half mile from Arrow Rock's Main Street and contains sites 13–47. All sites here are now electric, but many are still nice tenting spots. Sites 23–32 are closest to the restrooms and showers on a side loop off the main campground road. The only bad sites in this group are 24 and

:: Ratings

BEAUTY: ★ ★ ★
PRIVACY: ★ ★ ★
SPACIOUSNESS: ★ ★ ★
QUIET: ★ ★ ★ ★
SECURITY: ★ ★ ★ ★ ★
CLEANLINESS: ★ ★ ★ ★ ★

:: Key Information

ADDRESS: 39521 Visitor Center Dr. Arrow Rock, MO 65320

OPERATED BY: Missouri Department of Natural Resources

CONTACT: Park office, 660-837-3330; mostateparks.com/park/arrow-rock-state-historic-site

OPEN: Year-round, 7 a.m.–10 p.m.

SITES: 12 basic, 34 electric, 1 full hookup

SITE AMENITIES: Table, fire pit with grate, lantern pole

ASSIGNMENT: First come, first served; reservations at 877-ICAMPMO or park's website

REGISTRATION: Occupy site, pay host, or staff comes by to collect

FACILITIES: Apr. 15–Oct. 31: Showers, water, flush toilets, dump station; Year-round: Playground, visitor center, trails, historical sites

PARKING: At each site

FEE: Apr. 15–Oct. 31: $13 basic, $21 electric, $28 full hookup; Nov. 1–Apr. 14: $12 basic, $19 electric, $24 full hookup; $8.50 nonrefundable reservation fee; $2 discount for seniors and campers with disabilities

ELEVATION: 700'

RESTRICTIONS:

■ **Pets:** On 10-foot leash

■ **Fires:** In fire pits; campers must comply with current firewood advisories

■ **Alcohol:** Allowed in campsites but not in parking lots

■ **Vehicles:** Up to 60 feet

■ **Other:** 15-day camping limit; 6-person limit per site

26, jammed close together on the inside of the loop. The eight sites on the outside of the loop are spaced just right and have plenty of tent space. Site 28 at the end of the loop offers the most solitude. Sites 33–47 on the road east of the shower house contain many level sites, with site 38 at the road's end having the most privacy. The southern loop of this campground contains sites 13-22. Most sites on this loop are pull-through and thus attract bigger RVs, but sites 13, 15, 17, and 19 are nice back-in spots overlooking Big Soldier Lake.

The best place to begin your exploration of Arrow Rock is its superb visitor center. It's tucked away in a wooded hollow just south of Main Street so that its modern building won't detract from Arrow Rock's 19th-century architecture. It's one of the best visitor centers I've seen in a state park. Covering all the human history of the surrounding Boone's Lick country, it features American Indian artifacts; exhibits on the French and Spanish influence in central Missouri; information panels on the Louisiana Purchase, the Lewis and Clark Expedition, and the Santa Fe Trail; and other history of the territory around Arrow Rock. See gun and tool collections, admire several pieces of George Caleb Bingham's works, and view a 20-minute slide presentation on the history of Arrow Rock.

With its old storefronts, wooden sidewalks, and limestone gutters, Arrow Rock's Main Street truly is a trip into the past. One of the most interesting examples of Arrow Rock's 19th-century architecture is the Old Tavern, where you can take a tour and enjoy a meal. Founded in 1834 by Joseph Huston, it's thought to be the oldest continually operating restaurant west of the Mississippi River. Another interesting stop is the John P. Sites Pioneer Gun Shop, where for

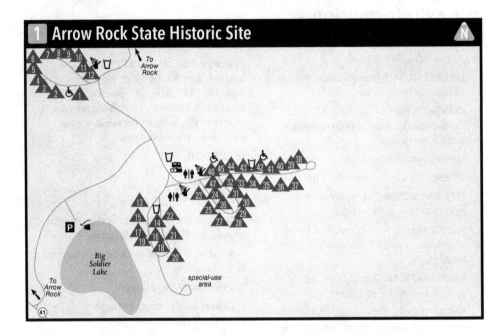

nearly 60 years in the late 1800s Mr. Sites built weapons for travelers headed for the Western frontier. The restored shop exhibits gunsmithing tools and several of John Sites's rare and valuable rifles. Take a walking tour of town to see more of Arrow Rock's 19th-century buildings, including the restored George Caleb Bingham house, the town doctor's home, the old courthouse, and the old stone jail. For a walk on the wilder side, head out on the Pierre a Flèche Trail, a 1.5-mile loop around the campground that visits a scenic overlook from the bluffs that gave Arrow Rock its name. When you're ready to sit for a while, visit the Lyceum Theater. During its five-month season the Lyceum features a variety of Broadway-style plays and musicals. Or browse Arrow Rock's several antiques and craft shops, and then rest your feet while dining in one of the town's four restaurants. Who would have thought camping could be so decadent?

:: Getting There

From Exit 98 on I-70, drive 13 miles north on MO 41. The campground entrance will be on the right just before you reach the town of Arrow Rock.

GPS COORDINATES   N 39° 3.795'   W 92° 56.785'

2

Cuivre River State Park

Cuivre River State Park's trails explore a landscape featuring clear streams, springs, bluff overlooks, and patches of tall-grass prairie.

Cuivre River State Park's 6,394 acres are an anomaly to the agricultural landscape around it, featuring the ridges, hollows, gravel-bottom streams, and bluff overlooks common to the Ozarks in the southern part of the state. It's part of the Lincoln Hills, an area that escaped the heavy glaciations of the lands around the park. Many plants and animals living here are found nowhere else in northern Missouri.

Cuivre River didn't become a park until 1946, but its construction got started in the 1930s as a federal demonstration project for the Civilian Conservation Corps and Works Progress Administration. As they did in so many parks and national forests in the Ozarks, these organizations built bridges, roads, group camps, and some of the excellent trail system that explores the Cuivre River's hills and hollows.

There's something for everyone at this attractive state park. Lincoln Lake, a 55-acre clear gem in the middle of the park, has a swimming beach, boat ramp, great fishing,

and a 4-mile lakeside trail. There are excellent picnic sites, shelters for reunions, and group camps for overnight get-togethers. An equestrian camp serves horse enthusiasts, and several of the park's trails are open for horseback riding. The diverse landscape in and around the park attracts a variety of wildlife, making it a great place for birders. Some 38 miles of trail meander through the park, exploring Big Sugar Creek Wild Area, North Woods Wild Area, and the Lincoln Hills Natural Area on loops ranging from 1 to 7 miles.

The campground accommodates everything from the single tent to the largest RV or horse trailer. Luckily, the horse camp is in a far corner of the park, and the RV sites are a good distance from the tent sites. The full-hookup sites are east of the campground entrance, laid out like a small city. The more laid-back and spacious part of the campground is west of the entrance, laid out in a Y-shaped configuration, with a side loop containing 15 electric sites. The remaining 5 of the camp's 19 electric sites are on the north side of the base of the Y.

The best tent sites are the basic camps on the arms of the Y. The northern arm has sites 25–37. Site 25, set back from the road a bit, is nice, but my favorite on this side of camp is site 35. It's on a long spur and well below road level, which makes it one of the more private spots. Site 30 on the turnaround

:: Ratings

BEAUTY: ★ ★ ★ ★
PRIVACY: ★ ★ ★
SPACIOUSNESS: ★ ★ ★ ★
QUIET: ★ ★ ★ ★
SECURITY: ★ ★ ★ ★ ★
CLEANLINESS: ★ ★ ★ ★ ★

:: Key Information

ADDRESS: 678 MO 147
Troy, MO 63379

OPERATED BY: Missouri Department
of Natural Resources

CONTACT: Park office, 636-528-7247;
mostateparks.com/park/cuivre-river-
state-park

OPEN: Apr. 15–Oct. 31, 6 a.m.–10 p.m.;
Nov. 1–Apr. 14, 7 a.m.–8 p.m.

SITES: 47 basic, 19 electric, 32 full
hookup, 14 equestrian electric

SITE AMENITIES: Table, fire pit with
grate, lantern pole

ASSIGNMENT: First come, first served;
reservations at 877-ICAMPMO or park's
website

REGISTRATION: Occupy site, pay host,
or staff comes by to collect

FACILITIES: Apr. 15–Oct. 31: Showers,
laundry, dump station; Year-round:
Water, pavilions, playground, visitor
center, trails

PARKING: At each site

FEE: Apr. 15–Oct. 31: $13 basic, $20
family basic, $21 electric, $36 family
electric, $28 full hookup; Nov. 1–
Apr. 14: $12 basic, $18 family basic, $19
electric, $32 family electric, $24 full
hookup; $8.50 nonrefundable reserva-
tion fee; $2 discount for seniors and
campers with disabilities

ELEVATION: 660'

RESTRICTIONS:

◼ **Pets:** On 10-foot leash

◼ **Fires:** In fire pits; campers must comply with current firewood advisories

◼ **Alcohol:** Allowed in campsites but
not on beaches, in parking lots, or in
public areas

◼ **Vehicles:** Up to 50 feet

◼ **Other:** 15-day camping limit; 6-person
limit per site; 2-night minimum stay for
weekend reservations

loop is a nice site with a view of the lake, but it's one of the park's two family sites.

The nicest basic sites are on the south arm of the Y, and to get one during the core summer months, you should make a reservation. My favorites are 46–49, walk-in sites on the turnaround loop. Spread well apart from one another, they're the most spacious and private sites here—yet they're close enough to the road that they're as convenient as car-camping sites. Site 50, located at the beginning of the turnaround loop, is also another decent site with good spacing around it. Most sites on the road leading to the turnaround loop are too close to the road for my taste. Exceptions are sites 41, 42, and 57. Their tent pads are a bit farther from the road than the others and have better spacing from their neighbors.

Once you've settled into camp, the visitor center is the place to start your exploration at Cuivre River State Park. There you'll find maps of the park and its trails, dates and times of interpretive hikes and nature walks, and schedules and subjects of upcoming programs in the campground's amphitheater. There are also fascinating displays of the park's history and prehistory, featuring both the CCC/WPA and American Indian activities in the park area. Excellent exhibits about the park's flora and fauna preview what you'll see in the park, and the center offers an excellent introductory slide show.

All the trails in Cuivre River are great hikes, but my favorites are the north half of the Lone Spring Trail and the western side of the Cuivre River Trail. The Cuivre River

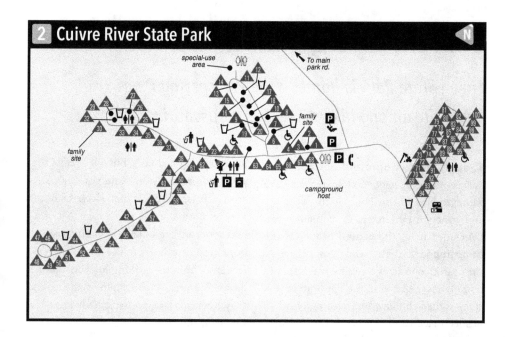

Trail is a 7-mile loop, with four connectors that let you shorten the hike as needed. Its west side follows Frenchman's Bluff for nearly 2 miles, with stunning views of the Cuivre River and its bottomland farms. For half of this stretch, the trail parallels a gravel road, and you'll have to share it with equestrians—but it's too pretty a hike to miss.

The Lone Spring Trail is less spectacular, but it's a wonderful hike on a smooth trail that's open to foot travel only. Its northern half wanders through the valleys and ridges of the upper forks of Big Sugar Creek. On the far western reaches of this trail, you'll see its namesake, Lone Spring, seeping gently from a low bluff.

:: Getting There

From Troy, drive 3 miles east to MO 147. Go left 2 miles on MO 147 to Lincoln Hills Road. Turn right and go 0.8 mile on Lincoln Hills to a four-way stop. Turn left, staying on Lincoln Hills Road, and go 1.6 miles to Mossy Hill Drive. Turn right and drive 1 mile on Mossy Hill Drive to the campground. Tent-camping sites are to the right at the campground entrance's T-intersection.

GPS COORDINATES   N 39° 1.844'   W 90° 54.625'

3

Hawn State Park

Hawn State Park is home to the Whispering Pines Trail,
a favorite among hikers in eastern Missouri.

Though the campground in Hawn State Park is more developed than most of the campgrounds in this book, with electricity and concrete parking pads at many sites, I included it for the natural beauty of the campground and the wild atmosphere of the nearly 5,000 acres contained in the park's boundaries. Located in the flat bottom of a steep-walled hollow, the campground is nestled in a meander of Pickle Creek. Hawn State Park is named for Helen Coffer Hawn, a teacher in nearby Ste. Genevieve, who in 1952 donated the park's first 1,459 acres. Her namesake park is a wonderful place to spend a few days relaxing in nature's splendor.

As you come down the hill from the park office, the picnic area and trailhead are to your right. Downhill another 100 yards the road ends in the campground. The first loop contains nine electric sites that are crowded just a little too close together. Just beyond that the main loop begins. The south half of the loop contains electric sites, while the north half has basic sites. Sites are spaced a little close together—close enough

to meet your neighbors, but not so tight that you'll get on each other's nerves. Basic sites are a little farther apart than electric sites, so they're more suitable for tenting. The best tent spots are the walk-in sites situated just beyond the north end of the loop. About 150 feet away from the parking lot, the walk-ins have more privacy and the best shade, and they are near a stream that's shaded by a low sandstone bluff.

Home to one of the most popular trails in Missouri, Hawn State Park is a hiker's dream. Whispering Pines Trail was built in the late 1970s with the help of the Sierra Club. This 10-mile loop is everything a trail should be. You'll wander through thick stands of the shortleaf pine forests that give the trail its name, meander along quiet streams, admire enchanting waterfalls and cascades, and be awed by spectacular vistas. One of these overlooks has two rock ledges that are the perfect places for a picnic with a view. Near its end the trail climbs to a bluff high above the campground, where you'll admire your campsite from the cliffs and anticipate enjoying a cold beverage at your picnic table after your hike.

The trail is divided into a 6-mile north loop and a 4-mile south loop. Other options are the 4-mile White Oak Trail and the 1-mile Pickle Creek Trail. The Pickle Creek Trail is spectacular, meandering past the most scenic spot in the park—the cascades, waterfalls, and shut-ins along Pickle Creek. It connects

:: Ratings

BEAUTY: ★ ★ ★ ★ ★
PRIVACY: ★ ★ ★
SPACIOUSNESS: ★ ★ ★ ★ ★
QUIET: ★ ★ ★ ★
SECURITY: ★ ★ ★ ★ ★
CLEANLINESS: ★ ★ ★ ★ ★

:: Key Information

ADDRESS: 12096 Park Dr.
Ste. Genevieve, MO 63670

OPERATED BY: Missouri Department
of Natural Resources

CONTACT: Park office, 573-883-3603;
mostateparks.com/park/hawn-state-park

OPEN: Mar. 15–Nov. 14, 7:30 a.m.–9 p.m.;
Nov. 15–Mar. 14, 7:30 a.m.–sunset

SITES: 19 basic, 26 electric, 5 walk-in,
3 with disabled access

SITE AMENITIES: Table, fire pit with
grate, lantern pole; some with tent pads

ASSIGNMENT: First come, first served;
reservations at 877-ICAMPMO or park's
website

REGISTRATION: Staff comes by to register and collect

FACILITIES: Apr.–Oct.: Water, showers,
flush toilets, laundry; Year-round: Phone,
amphitheater, picnic shelter, playground,
trails

PARKING: At each site

FEE: Apr.–Oct.: $13 basic, $21 electric;
Nov.–Mar.: $12 basic, $19 electric; $8.50
nonrefundable reservation; $2 discount
for seniors and campers with disabilities

ELEVATION: 580'

RESTRICTIONS:

■ **Pets:** On 10-foot leash

■ **Fires:** In fire pits; campers must comply with current firewood advisories

■ **Alcohol:** Allowed at campsites but not
in public areas

■ **Vehicles:** Up to 40 feet

■ **Other:** 15-day stay limit; 6-person limit
per site; 2-night minimum stay for weekend reservations Mar. 15–Nov. 14

with the northern segment of the Whispering Pines Trail, forming a 2-mile loop. If you
choose the Whispering Pines or Pickle Creek
Trails, plan for wet feet if you hike in spring
or after rain—both trails ford Pickle Creek at
least once. It's worth getting wet, though—the
heavier the stream flow, the more spectacular
the cascades, and during the Ozarks summer
heat and humidity, splashing through the
creek is an absolute delight.

Once you've hiked all the trails at Hawn,
go to the Pickle Springs Natural Area. Take
MO 32 a few miles west to MO AA, and then
go east 2 miles on MO AA to Dorlac Road.
Turn left on Dorlac and drive a half mile to
the parking area for the Trail Through Time.
This spectacular 2-mile loop, a designated
National Natural Landmark, is like a geological museum. If humans designed and built
a landscape like this one, we'd be accused
of exaggerating nature. Probably the most

fascinating 2-mile trek in the Ozarks, the
trail sports an incredible number of natural
marvels crammed in a 256-acre wonderland.
Best of all, it's an easy hike for novices, but
so fascinating that even hard-core trampers
will be enthralled.

The trail passes sandstone pillars that
look like they came from Utah's Bryce Canyon. You'll walk through the Slot, squeeze
through a narrow gap in the stone nick-
named the Keyhole, and admire Double
Arch, where two pillars support a huge sandstone ledge, forming the ideal shelter for a
rainy or hot and sunny day. Owl's Den Bluff
and Dome Rock overlooks give panoramic
views of the surrounding forest. Mossy Falls
comes to life when it rains, and another
small waterfall trickles off a small ledge near
Pickle Springs itself. Just past the springs
you'll come to Rockpile Canyon, where a
bluff collapse created an impressive rock

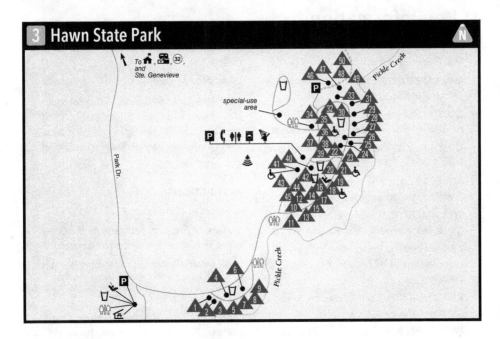

garden. If it has rained recently, Headwall Falls will be roaring into the canyon, and during cold snaps the falls are an incredible curtain of ice.

On all the trails in Hawn and Pickle Springs, you'll see plenty of wildflowers in spring; moss and ferns in the cool, moist areas sheltered by bluffs and rock ledges; and tremendous views from pine-studded cliffs. Bring your binoculars and bird guides when you come to Hawn State Park—many songbirds inhabit this diverse area, and you'll be lulled to sleep at night by the calls of owls and whippoorwills.

:: Getting There

From MO 32, exit off I-55 near Ste. Genevieve and drive west 12 miles to MO 144. Turn left (south) on MO 144 and follow it 4 miles to the park. Pass the park office, go down a long hill, and the road will end in the campground.

GPS COORDINATES   N 37° 49.959'   W 90° 13.596'

4

Johnson's Shut-Ins State Park

View the awesome power of runaway floodwaters from the Scour Trail, and then enjoy a relaxing splash in the Black River's cooling waterfalls and cascades.

Johnson's Shut-Ins, historically one of Missouri's most popular state parks, was almost completely destroyed in December 2005 by the blowout of nearby Taum Sauk Reservoir. Built to supply water for a nearby hydroelectric plant, this mountaintop lake burst its retaining wall and sent over a billion gallons roaring down the hillside to the Black River at Johnson's Shut-Ins. The flood devastated nearly all the park's facilities, including its riverside campground, in just a few minutes. Miraculously, no one was killed, but the park was closed for several years while it was cleaned up and rebuilt.

The resurrected version of Johnson's Shut-Ins features a beautiful new visitor center, more trails than ever, interpretive displays describing the flood and its effect on the area, and the park's favorite activity over the years—splashing in the shut-ins. With the reconstruction came a brand-new expanded campground. Located a couple of miles from the shut-ins by the Goggins Mountain Trailhead, it's connected to the

:: Ratings

BEAUTY: ★ ★ ★ ★ ★
PRIVACY: ★ ★
SPACIOUSNESS: ★ ★
QUIET: ★ ★ ★ ★
SECURITY: ★ ★ ★ ★ ★
CLEANLINESS: ★ ★ ★ ★ ★

park center by a paved biking-hiking trail. The new campground is much larger than the old camp and offers everything from basic sites to full hookups. It also includes showers and a shelter in each loop, an equestrian camp for horse lovers, cabins, and secluded walk-in sites. If you're planning a weekend visit to this popular park during the warm months, you'd better make reservations well in advance—it fills almost every weekend May–October.

The equestrian area is in the campground's first loop; it contains water and electric sites 101–110. Camping spots in this loop are not well shaded, but because they must accommodate horses and their trailers, they're the most spacious sites in the park. Loop 2 has full-hookup sites 201–220, overdeveloped camping spots geared more to large RVs. A spur road off Loop 2 leads to the park's camper cabins, six simply appointed hideaways for those who prefer to rough it smoothly. Sites 301–321 in Loop 3 are the campground's electric-only camping spots. With a couple of exceptions, sites on the loop's south side have space for tents, and those on the north half do not. Between Loops 2 and 3 you'll find the park store, with its playground, tables for hanging out and visiting, and Wi-Fi service to keep you in touch with the outside world.

Loop 4 holds the park's 14 basic park-in camping spots. The three sites inside the loop

:: Key Information

ADDRESS: 148 Taum Sauk Trl. Middlebrook, MO 63656

OPERATED BY: Missouri Department of Natural Resources

CONTACT: Park office, 573-546-2450; mostateparks.com/park/johnsons-shut-ins-state-park

OPEN: March 1–Wed. before Memorial Day and day after Labor Day–Oct. 31, 8 a.m.–6 p.m.; Thurs. before Memorial Day–Labor Day, 8 a.m.–7 p.m.; Nov.–Feb., 8 a.m.–4 p.m.; campground gates close at 10 p.m. Apr.–Oct.

SITES: 14 basic, 14 basic walk-in, 21 electric premium, 10 electric/water premium, 20 full hookup premium

SITE AMENITIES: table, lantern pole, fire pit with grill

ASSIGNMENT: First come, first served; reservations available, and highly recommended, Apr.–Oct. at 877-ICAMPMO or at park's website

REGISTRATION: At entrance check station; if closed, register at host site

FACILITIES: Apr.–Oct.: Water, dump station, laundry; Year-round: Showers, flush toilets, playground, visitor center, store with Wi-Fi

PARKING: At each site (except for walk-ins)

FEE: Apr.–Oct.: $13 basic, $23 electric premium, $25 electric/water premium, $28 full hookup premium; Nov.–Mar.: $12 basic, $21 electric premium and electric/water premium, $24 full hookup premium; $2 discount for seniors and campers with disabilities

ELEVATION: 880'

RESTRICTIONS

■ **Pets:** On 10-foot leash; not allowed in the shut-ins area

■ **Fires:** In fire rings; campers must comply with current firewood advisories

■ **Alcohol:** Allowed in campsites but not in parking lots and swimming areas

■ **Vehicles:** Up to 90 feet

■ **Other:** 15-day stay limit; 6-person limit per site; 4-person, 1-tent limit at walk-ins; 2-night minimum stay for weekend reservations Apr.–Oct.

road, close together with limited space suitable for tents, are the least attractive in Loop 4. Campsites along the outside of the loop are farther apart, much better shaded, and more spacious. The five outside sites on the loop's north side are the best—each is in a small alcove in the woods with shade, space, and more privacy. Sites 413 and 414 on the loop's south side are also very nice, but are close to the restrooms and their all-night lights.

The park's walk-in sites in Loop 5 require a little extra effort to reach, but they're well worth it if you like true solitude. Scattered along a wooded trail north and west of Loop 4, sites 501–514 are shady, secluded hideaways. Each has a wooden tent platform complete with table, lantern pole, and barbecue pit. Most of the tent platforms have railings too. Just bring some straps or rope for anchoring your tent to the platform, as well as gear bags that carry easily.

There's a lot to do at Johnson's Shut-Ins. After settling into camp, head for the Black River Center to get your bearings. There you'll find a gift shop; a small nature museum describing the flora, fauna, and geologic history of the area; brochures describing park activities; and trail maps that will show you the way through the surrounding backcountry.

Most folks visit the park for the Black River Shut-Ins. These waterfalls, cascades,

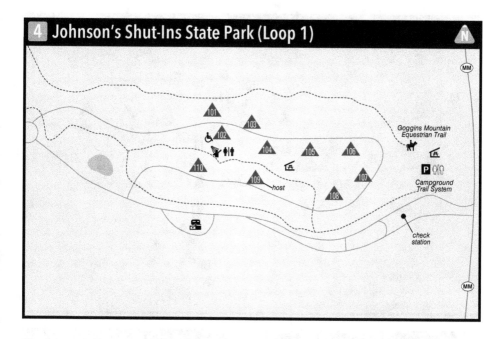

4 Johnson's Shut-Ins State Park (Loop 1)

(Map labels:) Goggins Mountain Equestrian Trail · Campground Trail System · host · check station

and chutes are a wonderful place to while away a hot summer day. You can wade in the shallows above the shut-ins, loll in the deep pool below them, or clamber onto the rugged expanse of volcanic rock that forms them to relax in your own favorite cascade, waterfall, or plunge pool. The number of visitors allowed in the shut-ins is limited on busy days, but campground users receive a special pass granting access at anytime.

The park's trails are a superb way to escape those crowds. The 2.25-mile Shut-Ins Trail takes you past the cascades to an overlook high above the stream, and then loops around to follow a ridge above the Black River back to the shut-ins parking area. If it has rained recently, there will be a waterfall at the loop's southern end, and a vista of the valley opens up just north of the falls. The 1.5-mile Horseshoe Glade Trail explores part of the East Fork Wild Area, passing through forest openings with views of the surrounding mountains. The 2-mile Scour Trail winds through the landscape destroyed

by the 2005 flood, showing both its devastation and nature's amazing power to regenerate itself. The park's longest hike, the Goggins Mountain Trail, starts right from Campground Loop 1 and wanders 10 miles along and over the shoulders of its namesake peak.

The Ozark Trail, Missouri's premier long-distance hiking route, links all four of these trails as it winds across Johnson's Shut-Ins. The OT's most popular section runs 13 miles from Johnson's Shut-Ins to Taum Sauk Mountain State Park (see page 37). It's a rugged up-and-down trek along the scenic backbone of Proffit Mountain, passing through the Devil's Toll Gate and over Mina Sauk Falls on its way to Missouri's highest point. Or get a ride to the shut-ins, and then combine the OT with segments of the Shut-Ins and Goggins Mountain Trails for an 11-mile trek back to the campground. Or just keep going north on the OT to the Bell Mountain Wilderness, Missouri's second-highest peak, and more vistas . . . the possibilities are almost endless at Johnson's Shut-Ins State Park!

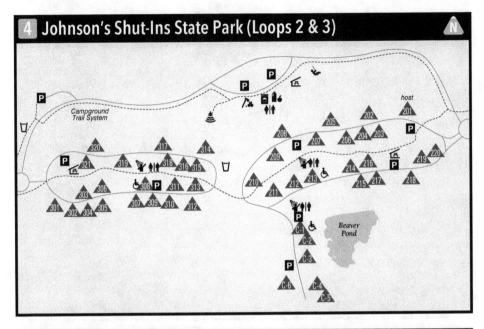

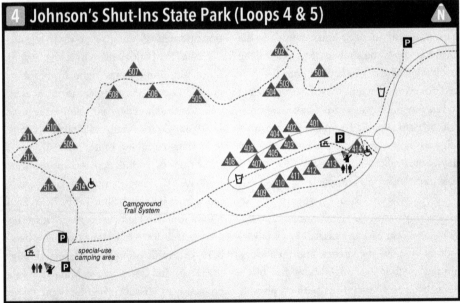

:: Getting There

From Potosi take MO 21 south 22 miles to MO N. Turn right and follow MO N 13 miles to MO MM. Turn right and drive 1 mile north to the campground entrance.

GPS COORDINATES N 37° 33.609' W 90° 51.086'

5

Klondike Park

Hike or mountain bike rugged trails, cycle along paved paths, or pedal the Katy Trail to wineries, restaurants, and shops in nearby Augusta and Defiance.

Klondike Park opened in 2004 on the site of the old Klondike Quarry. The quarry first opened in 1898, when the Tavern Rock Sand Company began crushing the park's sandstone to extract silica for making glass. After the quarry closed in 1983, nothing was done with the land for nearly 20 years, allowing this 250-acre work-scarred landscape to return to its natural beauty.

Now covered with hardwoods, cedars, a few pines, and lots of wildflowers and shrubs, the old quarry is a peaceful natural setting. An exquisite pool reflects the quarry bluffs in the center of the park, and another shallow pond in the park's north end is an attractive marsh and wetland that's excellent for bird-watching and wildflower-viewing. Five miles of trails meander through the park, and one path climbs to vistas of the Missouri River Valley. Klondike's trail system also connects to the 220-mile-long Katy Trail State Park, the longest rails-to-trails conversion in the country.

Klondike Park is an excellent place for group or family camping. Its 41 campsites

:: Ratings

BEAUTY: ★ ★ ★ ★ ★
PRIVACY: ★ ★
SPACIOUSNESS: ★ ★ ★
QUIET: ★ ★ ★
SECURITY: ★ ★ ★ ★ ★
CLEANLINESS: ★ ★ ★ ★ ★

are organized in four clusters, and six cabins are available for those in your crowd who don't want to rough it. There are 31 primitive campsites, simple camping spots with only a table and a grill, and 10 basic sites with table, grill, lantern pole, and table shelter. The basic sites are scattered farther apart than the primitive sites, so they offer more spaciousness and better privacy. A modern bathhouse is centrally located and comes complete with a small kitchen with deep sinks and a two-burner stove.

Primitive sites 1–10 are the first campsites you'll come to on the park's one-way loop road. Like all sites at Klondike, these are walk-in camping spots accessed by mulched trails. They're 30–60 yards from the parking area, scattered around a shady open space. A large pavilion in the campground makes an excellent escape during rainstorms. All sites are visible from one another, with site 6 at the back of the wooded enclave offering the most privacy.

Primitive sites 11–24 are north of sites 1–10 at the end of a spur road. Sites 11–15, located on the north and west sides of the parking area, are so close to the parking lot that they're like car-camping sites. They have a view of the wetland, with sites 11 and 14 offering the most privacy. Sites 16–24 are east of the parking area, in a grassy opening in the woods. While all nine of these sites are good tenting spots with level grass and

:: Key Information

ADDRESS: 4600 MO 94 S.
Augusta, MO 63332

OPERATED BY: St. Charles County Parks
Department

CONTACT: 636-949-7535;
parks.sccmo.org

OPEN: Year-round, 7 a.m.–30 minutes
after sunset

SITES: 31 primitive, 10 basic; all are
walk-in

SITE AMENITIES: Table, fire ring with
grill; basic sites have lantern pole, tent
pad, sheltered table

ASSIGNMENT: First come, first served;
reservations accepted by phone

REGISTRATION: By reservation or self-
register at pay station by bathhouse

FACILITIES: Apr.–Oct.: Water, showers,
flush toilets; Year-round: Composting
toilets, picnic areas, pavilions, trails,
playgrounds, cabins, conference center

PARKING: At parking lot adjacent to sites

FEE: $7 primitive, $10 basic

ELEVATION: 500'

RESTRICTIONS:

- **Pets:** On 8-foot leash
- **Fires:** In fire rings
- **Alcohol:** In manufactured-sealed con-
tainers with 5% or less alcohol content
- **Vehicles:** Car length
- **Other:** 15-day stay limit; 5-person,
2-tent limit per site; no rock climbing;
no glass containers

some shade, they're just a bit too close to MO 94 for true peace and quiet.

Primitive sites 25–31 are south of the picnic area, close to the Katy Trail access path. Sites 25–28 are hidden away among boulders next to a rock wall left over from the quarry operation. Sites 25, 26, and 27 are tight, open, and exposed, but are great spots for fall or winter camping. Site 28 is excellent, tucked back in the trees with space for a couple of tents. Sites 29, 30, and 31 are on a small hill above site 28. With lots of space around it, site 30 is the best of these three well-shaded sites.

My favorite sites at Klondike Park are in the 10-site basic campground. They're farther apart than most of the primitive sites and more spacious, and each one has a table shelter, guaranteeing you at least a little shade. Except for site 1, an accessible camping spot, all are comfortably far from the road, and the bathhouse is only a few steps away. Sites 3 and 4 are nice spots off

by themselves at the west end of the basic camp, directly across from the showers. At the east end of this camp are sites 9 and 10, another pair of camping spots off by themselves. Sites 2, 6, 7, and 8 in the middle of camp are decent campsites, but are a bit close to each other. The best spot in the basic campground is site 5. It's located at the end of a shady little cove in the trees, with woods on three sides.

Don't miss the activities in and around the park. Visitors can explore the park on foot or from the seat of a mountain bike on 1 mile of paved trail and 4 miles of natural surface paths. One of these, the 2-mile Hogsback Trail, climbs to an incredible overlook of the Missouri River Valley. Two additional nearby trails, both open to hikers and bikers, are the 3-mile Matson Hill Trail and the 8-mile Lost Valley Trail. Another superb trail, open to foot traffic only, is the Lewis and Clark Trail. This 8-mile loop goes to several vistas of the Missouri River as it winds through the

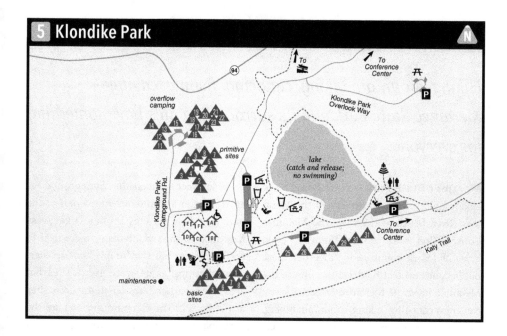

5 Klondike Park

Weldon Spring Wildlife Area. The Lewis and Clark and Lost Valley Trails are on MO 94 north of Defiance, and the Matson Hill Trail is just east of Matson Hill.

To combine exercise with the finer things in life, hike or bike the Katy Trail to the nearby towns of Defiance, Augusta, Dutzow, and Marthasville. In these quaint villages, founded by Germans in the 1800s, you'll find wineries, a microbrewery, restaurants, shops, and bike rentals. And though it's not on the Katy Trail, don't miss Montelle Winery with its bluff-top views. It's on MO 94 at the top of Klondike Hill, just west of the park.

:: Getting There

From I-64/US 40, take Exit 10 for Weldon Spring, Defiance, and MO 94. Drive south 14 miles on MO 94 to Klondike Park on the left side of the highway.

GPS COORDINATES   N 38° 34.799'   W 90° 50.450'

6

Meramec State Park

Hiking, mountain biking, canoeing, fishing, caving—
Meramec State Park and its surrounding hills have something
for everyone.

Meramec State Park covers 6,800 acres of wooded hills on the north side of the Meramec River. South of the river, the Meramec Conservation Area contains another 3,900 acres of Ozark countryside. Together these public lands protect 8 attractive miles of the Meramec River. At Meramec State Park you can enjoy canoeing, hiking, mountain biking, fishing, and even exploring the Ozarks underground in one of the park's numerous caves.

Like many Missouri state parks, Meramec is somewhat overdeveloped. Over the last few years many once-basic sites have become wired for electricity. Still, Meramec State Park is so attractive that I included it anyway. It has something for everyone. If you don't feel like cooking, head over to the Fireside Grill. A noncamper who wants to spend the weekend with you can rent one of the park's cabins and meet you for hikes, canoeing, or other activities in the park. At the park entrance there's an excellent visitor center with information and exhibits on the park's trails, geology, and wildlife.

:: Ratings

BEAUTY: ★ ★ ★ ★ ★
PRIVACY: ★ ★
SPACIOUSNESS: ★ ★ ★ ★
QUIET: ★ ★ ★ ★
SECURITY: ★ ★ ★ ★
CLEANLINESS: ★ ★ ★ ★ ★

Meramec's riverside campground is at the east end of the developed part of the park. The first 179 sites are in a large grassy field next to the river. Sites 1–20 are next to the Meramec, but they're full-hookup sites. Most of campsites 21–59 are electric sites that are close together. Sites 60–111 are basic sites at the back of the campground and are the best spaced and quietest camping spots in the main campground. Sites 112–177 in the north end of the campground are on a triangular field between the river and a bluff, shaded by massive oaks; all these sites are now electric, and 112–125 have water hookups.

Don't be discouraged with this huge campground—the best tent sites are ahead. Follow the camp's main road as it curves around and doubles back along the river past the full-hookup campsites. Just when you think you're leaving the park, you'll find two loops with great tent camping. The first of these tent loops contains sites 181–188. The sites are level, grassy, and spacious, but some are close to the road. They all have electricity, and a few have water hookups, but are still nicer than sites in the main campground.

The second loop is where you'll find the best camping spots. Sites 189–210 are in a shady hollow next to the Meramec River, with a pretty bluff overlooking the river to the south. The openness of the loop means minimal privacy, but its sites are level and shady, have room for two tents, and, although they

:: Key Information

ADDRESS: 115 Meramec Park Dr. Sullivan, MO 63080

OPERATED BY: Missouri Department of Natural Resources

CONTACT: Park office, 573-468-6072; mostateparks.com/park/meramec-state-park

OPEN: Apr.-Oct., 7 a.m.-10 p.m.; Nov.-March, 7 a.m.-9 p.m.

SITES: 50 basic, 124 electric, 14 electric/water, 24 full hookup, 3 group

SITE AMENITIES: Table, fire pit with grate, lantern pole

ASSIGNMENT: First come, first served; reservations at 877-ICAMPMO or park's website

REGISTRATION: Occupy site, register and pay at entrance

FACILITIES: Apr.-Oct.: Showers, flush toilets, laundry, dump station; Year-round: Water, vault toilets, visitor center, restaurant, cabins, store, conference center, picnic area, canoe rentals, trails

PARKING: At each site

FEE: Apr.-Oct.: $13 basic, $23 electric, $25 electric/water, $28 full hookup; Nov.-Mar.: $12 basic, $21 electric and electric/water, $24 full hookup; $8.50 nonrefundable reservation fee; $2 discount for seniors and campers with disabilities

ELEVATION: 580'

RESTRICTIONS:
■ **Pets:** On 10-foot leash
■ **Fires:** In fire pits; campers must comply with current firewood advisories
■ **Alcohol:** Allowed in campsites but not in parking lots or swimming areas
■ **Vehicles:** Up to 40 feet
■ **Other:** 15-day stay limit; 6-person limit per site; 2-night minimum stay for weekend reservations

seem remote, are actually the most centrally located campsites in the park. Though they're electric sites, the small size of their parking spaces will keep the bigger RVs away. Sites 189–210 are closed during the off-season.

At the far end of the campground road are three group camps. For a camping party with your family or friends, these sites can't be beat. They're among the best group sites I've ever seen. They're remote, heavily shaded, next to the river, and close to the showers.

The 60 miles of the Meramec River from Meramec Spring to Meramec State Park offer some of the most beautiful canoeing in Missouri. Canoe rentals are available in the park and from outfitters located up and down the Meramec. They'll set you up for single- or multiday floats ending at your campsite in the park. You'll drift past wooded hills, farms, springs, and picturesque bluffs.

One of those bluffs towers over Green's Cave, 5 miles upstream from the campground. In my opinion, this is the prettiest place in the park. It's an easy climb to the top of the bluff to enjoy a panoramic vista of the river and fields below. Beneath you, a huge cavern is hollowed out of the bluff, with a cave and spring pouring out of the bluff's back. Squeezing a few feet into the cave, you enter a large subterranean room.

You could explore farther into Green's Cave, but don't take that risk unless you're with experienced spelunkers. For a safe cave experience, go back to the park's center and tour Fisher Cave. Located next to the campground, Fisher Cave can be explored by a mile-long guided underground hike. (To slow the spread of white nose fungus among Missouri's bat population, Fisher Cave was closed indefinitely in 2013. It should reopen in future

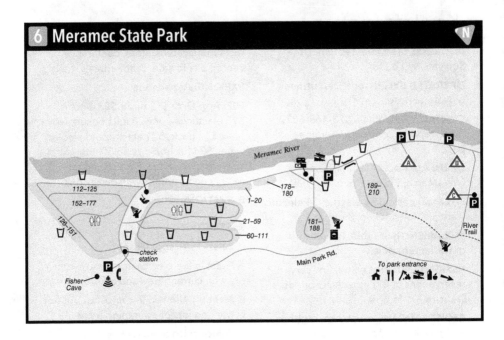

6 Meramec State Park

Meramec River

112–125

152–177

126–151

check station

Fisher Cave

178–180

1–20

21–59

60–111

181–188

189–210

River Trail

Main Park Rd.

To park entrance

years, but you can still do a little spelunking right now by heading west about 20 miles to Onondaga Cave State Park near Leasburg, and taking an underground tour there.)

The park's 16 miles of hiking trails are a wonderful introduction to the Ozarks hills and forests. Bluff View Trail showcases incredible vistas of the river valley. River Trail is an easy hike along the Meramec, where you're likely to spot kingfishers and herons along the river. The 10-mile Wilderness Trail has a 6-mile southern loop and a 4-mile northern loop, with overnight camps for backpackers. You'll see several of the park's caves on your hikes along its trail system.

Across the river in Meramec Conservation Area, there's a mountain bike trail suitable for cyclists of all skill levels. This 12-mile, two-loop trail system follows old logging roads and abandoned doubletracks through forested hills south of the river. There's also an 8-mile hiking trail in the conservation area. Both trails pass the Old Reedville School site. Marked only by a stone and a couple of logs, the site is a fascinating reminder of days gone by on the Meramec.

On your drive to the conservation area, watch for an unmarked turnout on the left side of MO 185 just as you top the climb from the river valley. From this spot, a short interpretive trail explores what's left of a Civilian Conservation Corps camp. Only scattered foundations and three weathered stone chimneys remain to tell the story of CCC Company 2728's work in the surrounding forest between 1934 and 1942.

:: Getting There

Drive 3 miles south of Sullivan on MO 185. Turn right into the park and follow signs to the campground.

GPS Coordinates   N 38° 12.456'   W 91° 6.127'

7

St. Francois State Park

Explore Mooner's Hollow on a trail named for whiskey makers who once worked their stills along scenic Coonville Creek.

"Yesterday's Hideout, Today's Retreat," St. Francois State Park's motto, evokes the legend that Civil War outlaws took cover in the hills and hollows that now make up the park. Later, moonshiners worked their stills in the narrow and scenic hollow along the banks of Coonville Creek, a place now preserved in the park's Coonville Creek Wild Area. In the early 1960s, hoping to preserve part of their landscape in its natural state, the residents of St. Francois County ran a door-to-door campaign for donations to buy land for the proposed park. From their first acreage purchase in 1964, St. Francois State Park has grown to its current 2,735 acres. Now it's a beautiful hideaway with attractive campgrounds, picnic sites, trails, and overlooks of the Big River.

The campground is located at the far end of the park road, nestled in a bend of the Big River. The lower campground features electric sites 1–63, and though it's a pretty area, it's a place tent campers should avoid. Its sites are too close together, and on nice weekends it's wall-to-wall RVs. Instead, take the left fork as you enter the campground and

:: Ratings

BEAUTY: ★ ★ ★ ★
PRIVACY: ★ ★
SPACIOUSNESS: ★ ★ ★
QUIET: ★ ★ ★ ★
SECURITY: ★ ★ ★ ★ ★
CLEANLINESS: ★ ★ ★ ★ ★

check out the park's 46 basic sites. Scattered along two loops laid out in the shape of a barbell, the basic sites at St. Francois State Park are more spacious, farther apart, and just as shady as the electric sites down by the river. Best of all, even on busy weekends, when the electric campground fills, you won't usually be crowded in the basic campsite loop.

Campers will find 11 sites in the first loop of the basic campground, and these are the places to be if you like being near the action. They're near the bathhouse, amphitheater, and trailheads for the hikes leading from the campground, and with a small playground located in the loop, they're good for families. Site 70, on the outside of the loop, off by itself and shaded by pines, is the best site on this end of the barbell. Sites 66 and 67 on the inside of the loop are nice and roomy, but very open and only partially shaded. The others on this first loop are only average at best.

The north loop of the basic campground, where you'll find sites 71–106, offers the most secluded camping in St. Francois State Park. It's farthest from the restrooms and other amenities, so fewer people go back there. The east side of the loop, with sites 71–88, has the best campsites. With a few exceptions, they're well spaced and roomy, and many are shaded by pines. Sites 71–79 on the first part of the loop are the best for shade and spacing. Though site 79 is a bit tight, you can fit your tent into a cedar

:: Key Information

ADDRESS: 8920 US 67 N.
Bonne Terre, MO 63628

OPERATED BY: Missouri Department
of Natural Resources

CONTACT: Park office, 573-358-2173;
mostateparks.com/park/st-francois-
state-park

OPEN: Apr.-Oct., 7 a.m.-10 p.m.;
Nov.-Mar., 8 a.m.-6 p.m.

SITES: 46 basic, 63 electric

SITE AMENITIES: Table, fire pit with
grate, lantern pole

ASSIGNMENT: First come, first served;
reservations at 877-ICAMPMO or park's
website

REGISTRATION: On summer weekends
register at entrance; on weekdays select
site and host will collect; Nov.-Mar., self-
pay at entrance booth

FACILITIES: Apr.-Oct.: Water, showers,

laundry, dump station; Year-round: Pavilions, amphitheater, playground, trails

PARKING: At each site

FEE: Apr.-Oct.: $13 basic, $20 family
basic, $21 electric; Nov.-Mar.: $12 basic,
$18 family basic, $19 electric; $8.50 non-
refundable reservation fee; $2 discount
for seniors and campers with disabilities

ELEVATION: 660'

RESTRICTIONS:

■ **Pets:** On 10-foot leash

■ **Fires:** In fire pits; campers must comply with current firewood advisories

■ **Alcohol:** Allowed in campsites but not
in parking lots or riverside

■ **Vehicles:** Electric sites, up to 70 feet;
basic sites, 20-40 feet

■ **Other:** 15-day stay limit; 6-person
limit per site; 2-night minimum stay for
weekend reservations

---

grove behind the site if it's not too big. Sites 89–106 on the west side are decent places to camp in a pinch, but are crowded a bit too close together for comfort.

St. Francois is a great park for hiking. Four trails covering 17 miles explore the park. The 11-mile Pike Run Trail is the longest hike at St. Francois. Divided into two loops of 7 and 4 miles each, it's popular with equestrians and is a pretty good place for trail runners and folks looking for an all-day hike.

The half-mile Missouri Trail and the 2.7-mile Swimming Deer Trail start from the campground loops. The Missouri Trail starts behind the bathhouse and runs behind the electric loops to the Big River, crossing the Swimming Deer Trail along the way. Just before ending on a gravel bar next to the river, it passes some monstrous

250-year-old sycamores. I once heard that early pioneers hollowed out river-bottom sycamores and lived in them, and after seeing the largest of these behemoths, I can believe it.

The Swimming Deer Trail is really a nice one. It starts from the end of the electric campsites and winds through moist bottomlands for a while, and then climbs onto a bluff with a couple of spectacular overlooks of the Big River streaming by below. Soon after leaving the overlooks the trail arcs away from the bluff, and on the way back to camp it wanders through rock gardens, goes by an abandoned barn left over from the area's pre-park days, and passes the sinkhole-like cave entrance. The cave is fenced off, but it's interesting to peer down into the earth's cooling breath emanating from the cave.

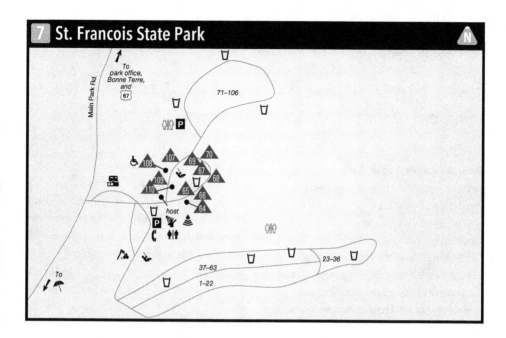

7 St. Francois State Park

The best hike at St. Francois State Park is the 2.7-mile Mooner's Hollow Trail. It explores both sides of the narrow valley of Coonville Creek, where the moonshiners once distilled white lightning. For a mile or so the trail follows this pretty creek (its waters were once part of the whiskey-making process), sometimes alongside its banks and other times on ledges above the stream. Huge mossy rocks cover the slopes above the creek bottom, and the trail winds over and through them. It crosses the creek near a long reflecting pool, complete with rocks to sit on while enjoying the scene, and then loops back to the trailhead through the hills on the west side of Coonville Creek.

:: Getting There

St. Francois State Park is located 4 miles north of Bonne Terre on the east side of US 67. Look for large brown signs at the entrance. The campground is at the end of the park road, next to the Big River.

GPS COORDINATES   N 37° 57.347'   W 90° 32.006'

8

Sam A. Baker State Park

Sam A. Baker State Park is nestled in the St. Francois Mountains, one of the oldest mountain ranges in North America.

Sam A. Baker State Park is named for a past governor of Missouri who was born in the area and pushed for the park's creation while he was in office in the mid-1920s. His namesake park, one of Missouri's oldest, is located in rugged mountains dating back to Precambrian times. When the surrounding St. Francois Mountains were formed, volcanoes dominated the landscape. Nowadays you can camp, hike, canoe, bicycle, or just hang out in the craggy forested hills where ash and lava once ruled.

All the development in this 5,164-acre state park is confined to the park's center along MO 143. The rest of Sam A. Baker State Park remains wild and unspoiled. Even the developed central corridor is a pretty place. The dining room, cabins, and three trail shelters were built by the Civilian Conservation Corps in the 1930s, and the grounds are beautifully landscaped and maintained.

Most of Sam A. Baker's campsites are in two campgrounds connected by a paved bike trail running through both camps to the park store. An additional 21 sites are in the Equestrian Campground across Big Creek from the

:: Ratings

BEAUTY: ★ ★ ★ ★ ★
PRIVACY: ★ ★ ★
SPACIOUSNESS: ★ ★ ★ ★
QUIET: ★ ★ ★ ★
SECURITY: ★ ★ ★ ★ ★
CLEANLINESS: ★ ★ ★ ★ ★

rest of the park. Campground 1, with sites 1–95 and 195–207, is a mile south of the park center. Sites here aren't far apart, but most are level, spacious, and shaded by groves of pines and hardwoods. The loop with sites 1–39 contains a mix of basic, electric, and family sites. Campsites 40–73 are tightly spaced electric sites not good for tent campers. The spur with basic sites 74–95 has the most spacious campsites, with sites 80–89 at the end of the road being the most secluded. Sites 195–207 are a loop of nicely spaced and shaded electric sites at the camp's north end. Although many sites in Campground 1 offer only limited privacy, its remote location makes it the more peaceful of Sam A. Baker's two campgrounds.

Campground 2 is a barbell-shaped loop of 80 campsites just south of the park center. All but nine of its sites are electric and spacing is tight, but its shady and pretty setting along the banks of Big Creek make it a pretty nice place to camp anyway. Campground 2's best tent sites are at its south end, where basic sites 155–160 are scattered along a short dead-end spur. Though the sites in Campground 2 are closer together and less private than the sites in Campground 1, many people prefer them for their pretty setting near the park's amenities.

Sam A. Baker is a great place for horse enthusiasts. Its 21-site equestrian camp is the perfect spot to hang out before and after a horseback jaunt through the mountains on the Mudlick Trail. It has 10 electric sites and

:: Key Information

ADDRESS: Route 1, Box 18150 Patterson, MO 63956

OPERATED BY: Missouri Department of Natural Resources

CONTACT: Park office, 573-856-4411; mostateparks.com/park/sam-baker-state-park

OPEN: Year-round, 7 a.m.–10 p.m.

SITES: 52 basic, 3 family basic, 136 electric, 9 family electric

SITE AMENITIES: Table, fire pit with grate, lantern pole

ASSIGNMENT: First come, first served; reservations at 877-ICAMPMO or park's website

REGISTRATION: Apr.–Oct., occupy site, register at camp fee office; Nov.–Mar., staff comes by site to collect

FACILITIES: Apr.–Oct.: Water, flush toilets, showers, laundry, dump station; Year-round: Vault toilets, picnic area, pavilions, store, dining room, cabins, nature center, playgrounds, river, canoe rental, trails

PARKING: At each site, on pavement

FEE: Apr.–Oct.: $13 basic, $26 family basic, $21 electric, $42 family electric, $23 electric premium, $46 family electric premium; Nov.–Mar.: $12 basic, $24 family basic, $19 electric, $38 family electric, $21 electric premium, $42 family electric premium; $8.50 nonrefundable reservation fee; $2 discount for seniors and campers with disabilities

ELEVATION: 420'

RESTRICTIONS:

■ **Pets:** On 10-foot leash

■ **Fires:** In fire pits; campers must comply with current firewood advisories

■ **Alcohol:** Allowed at campsites but not in public areas

■ **Vehicles:** Up to 50 feet

■ **Other:** 15-day stay limit; 2-night minimum stay for weekend and holiday reservations May 15–Sept. 15

---

11 basic ones, all with hitching posts and long parking pads for horse trailers. A trailhead for the Mudlick Trail is located in the Equestrian Campground. (You must be camping with horses to use the equestrian loop.)

Stop at Sam A. Baker's visitor center to acquaint yourself with the landscape's flora, fauna, and geology before exploring the park. The center has live snakes and turtles in terrariums, skulls, rock samples, and stuffed animals, including owls and hawks. During the park's busy season, interpretive talks and hikes are weekly features. The nature center's hours vary through the year, so check the park's website to make sure it will be open while you're at the park.

Just north of the visitor center is Sam A. Baker's picturesque dining hall. Showcasing the impressive stone-and-log construction of 1930s-vintage CCC architecture, it's a wonderful place to enjoy a delicious meal. Perched on the bank of Big Creek, the dining hall sports a vista of the stream from the big windows on the east wall. The dining hall is a great amenity for those who go camping to get away from mundane cooking chores, and its excellent dishes are a nice contrast to roughing it in your campsite.

In spring Big Creek is perfect for wading, swimming, tubing, or canoeing. The Shut-Ins Trail leads 1 mile upstream from the dining hall to a nice swimming hole among rocky outcrops in Big Creek. The St. Francis River meanders past the southeast part of the park near Campground 1 and is a good float year-round. The St. Francis is a raging whitewater river far upstream at Silver Mines, but by the time it reaches Sam A. Baker it's a placid

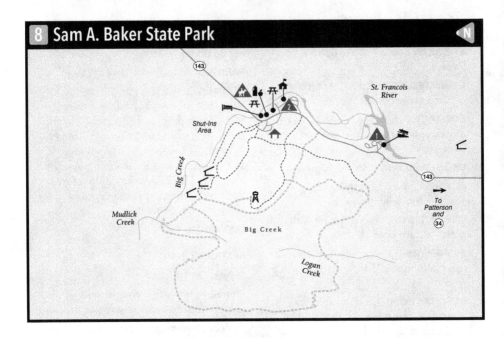

8 | Sam A. Baker State Park

float all the way to Lake Wappapello. In these pretty streams, you can fish for bass, bluegill, sunfish, goggle-eye, crappie, and catfish. Canoes and tubes for exploring both streams can be rented in the park.

You can explore the park's backcountry on the Mudlick Mountain National Recreation Trail, a 14-mile network of paths wandering through the landscape around Mudlick Mountain and Big and Logan Creeks. A spur leads to 1,313-foot Mudlick Mountain, where a fire tower stands in a grove of whispering pines. Highlights of this hike are three CCC-constructed stone trail shelters along the network's northeast side. These 80-year-old stone-and-log structures

look like part of the landscape. Even if you're not a hiker, summon the energy to hike the mile from the lodge to the first shelter. It's crouched on the lip of a bluff overlooking Big Creek, with spectacular views of the stream's steep-walled valley.

Miles of mountain biking await you at Sam A. Baker. Just south of Campground 1 is a trailhead for the Ozark Trail. From there, the Lake Wappapello Section of the Ozark Trail meanders 31 miles to MO 172, often skirting the shores of its namesake lake. At its south end this trail connects to the Lake Wappapello Trail, totaling more than 40 miles of scenic Ozark mountain biking.

:: Getting There

From Patterson on MO 34, drive 4 miles north on MO 143 to Sam A. Baker State Park. You'll come to Campground 1 first and then reach Campground 2.

GPS COORDINATES   N 37° 15.434'   W 90° 30.255'

9

Taum Sauk Mountain State Park

At 1,772 feet, Taum Sauk Mountain State Park is the highest point in Missouri.

With 7,500 acres in the rocky, rugged St. Francois Mountains, Taum Sauk Mountain State Park, the highest point in the state, is one of Missouri's newest and most scenic parks. This primitive, quiet campground is situated a few hundred yards from the High Point on a fairly flat part of the rounded top of the mountain. Far from any major city and at the end of a dead-end highway, Taum Sauk Mountain State Park's campground is remote and peaceful. Unlike most state parks, the campground is undeveloped, uncrowded, and rustic: in other words, ideal for tent campers.

All of Taum Sauk Mountain State Park's 12 sites are walk-in, but because the distance from the parking areas is only 25–50 feet, it's almost like a park-in campsite. Each parking area serves two or three sites, which are angled away from each other to provide good spacing. These shaded and level sites are scattered along a spur off the park road, and a scout camp available for groups is located at the end of the road. Restrooms

:: Ratings

BEAUTY: ★ ★ ★ ★ ★
PRIVACY: ★ ★ ★
SPACIOUSNESS: ★ ★ ★ ★ ★
QUIET: ★ ★ ★ ★ ★
SECURITY: ★ ★ ★
CLEANLINESS: ★ ★ ★ ★ ★

and water are located at the beginning of the campground road, near the picnic area and pay station. Site 1 is accessible. Also, because campsites at Taum Sauk are level with gravel paths leading from parking areas, most could serve campers with all but the most serious accessibility issues.

The park road ends a quarter mile past the campground entrance, at the parking lot for the High Point. Here you'll find more restrooms and a signboard with maps and information on the park and surrounding area. A short walk on a level concrete sidewalk leads to a marker for the highest point in Missouri.

Near the marker begins the attraction that brings most visitors to this mountaintop getaway—a spur leading to the Mina Sauk Falls Trail. This 3-mile loop descends Taum Sauk Mountain and opens up panoramic views of the surrounding countryside as you travel down to the Ozark Trail junction. After hiking 1 mile down the mountain, you'll join the Ozark Trail at Mina Sauk Falls, a 132-foot cascade that is the highest waterfall in Missouri. The falls are truly impressive in spring, when plenty of water splashes over the rocks. I like the Mina Sauk Falls Loop best in winter, when ice sculptures form on the boulders and pools that make up the cascade. Whatever time you visit the park, Mina Sauk Falls is one of the most entrancing sites in the state.

:: Key Information

ADDRESS: 148 Taum Sauk Trl. Middlebrook, MO 63656

OPERATED BY: Missouri Department of Natural Resources

CONTACT: Park office, 573-546-2450; mostateparks.com/park/taum-sauk-mountain-state-park

OPEN: Year-round

SITES: 12

SITE AMENITIES: Table, fire pit with grate, lantern pole

ASSIGNMENT: First come, first served

REGISTRATION Self-pay at entrance

FACILITIES: Apr.–Oct.: Water; Year-round: Vault toilets, trails, picnic areas

PARKING: Next to site, walk-in 25–50 feet

FEE: Apr.–Oct.: $13; Nov.–Mar.: $12; $2 discount for seniors and campers with disabilities

ELEVATION: 1,700'

RESTRICTIONS:

■ **Pets:** On 10-foot leash

■ **Fires:** In fire pits; campers must comply with current firewood advisories

■ **Alcohol:** Allowed at campsites but not in public areas

■ **Vehicles:** No length limit; tent camping only; pop-up or other trailers not allowed

■ **Other:** 15-day stay limit; 6-person limit per site

For even more spectacular scenery, continue west on the Ozark Trail. A mile west of the falls you'll pass through Devil's Toll Gate. Here the trail slips through an 8-foot gap in a rock 50 feet long and 30 feet high. An old wagon road following this narrow valley had to go through the tollgate. The wagons were unloaded, turned on their sides to fit through Devil's Toll Gate, and then reloaded before continuing down the rugged road.

For additional views, bring your backpack or arrange a shuttle, and hike the Ozark Trail 13 miles from Taum Sauk to Johnson's Shut-Ins State Park. Along the way you'll pass through open hillside glades with beautiful mountain vistas. I like hiking the long spine of Proffit Mountain, where mountain breezes cool me and ridgetop views awe me, especially in fall and winter, when the leaves are off the trees. Don't forget your hiking boots—this section of the Ozark Trail is very rugged, and sneakers won't cut it.

If you get a little worn down, no problem—the perfect anodyne awaits you at the end of the trail. You can cool those aching feet and sore muscles in the swimming holes, cascades, and fast-flowing chutes at Johnson Shut-Ins, where the east fork of the Black River flows over fantastic rock formations in this otherworldly state park. For climbers, several good routes can be found up the steep rock faces beneath the overlooks above Johnson's Shut-Ins. (Climbing is only allowed during certain months, and a permit is required. Check at the Johnson's Shut-Ins visitor center before you climb.) After your swim or climb, take a shower, get a cold drink and snack at the park store, and explore the park's superb new visitor center before heading back to the quieter, more remote Taum Sauk Mountain.

Once back at Taum Sauk Mountain State Park, grab your binoculars and climb the lookout tower to admire the terrain you just covered. Located on Department of Conservation land near the park entrance, the lookout opens up a 360-degree view of the St. Francois Mountains. The lookout

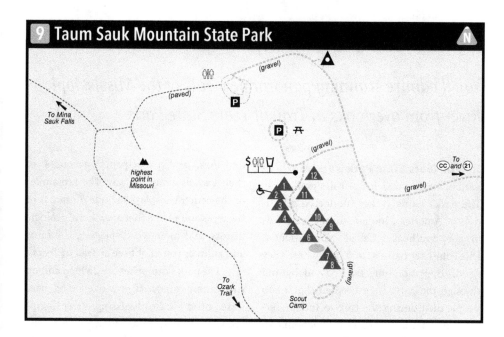

9 Taum Sauk Mountain State Park

(gravel)

(paved)

To Mina
Sauk Falls

highest
point in
Missouri

To
CC and 21

(gravel)

(gravel)

To
Ozark
Trail

Scout
Camp

(gravel)

---

shack on top is usually locked, but you can climb nearly to the top of the tower and take in the surrounding countryside. The view is especially spectacular at sunrise, when the area opens, and sunset, as the site is closing.

One of the more interesting landscape features visible from the lookout is the Upper Reservoir of Taum Sauk Mountain Hydroelectric Plant. What looks like a flat-topped peak is actually a man-made mountaintop lake used to generate power for the surrounding communities. In December 2005 this reservoir breached, sending 1.3 billion gallons of water roaring down the mountainside to the Black River. Miraculously, no

one was killed, but the cascade devastated nearby Johnson's Shut-Ins State Park. If you do the previously mentioned hike from Taum Sauk to Johnson's Shut-Ins, you'll trek right through the blowout's destruction as you approach the Black River (see page 21).

When camping on Missouri's highest point, plan some after-dinner stargazing from the mountaintop. Far from intrusive city lights and high above the surrounding countryside, Taum Sauk offers amazing vistas of night skies, especially on cold winter nights that freeze the moisture from the sky.

:: Getting There

From Ironton drive south 5 miles on MO 21/72 to MO CC. Turn right onto MO CC and go 4 miles to the park. The campground is 0.75 mile beyond where the pavement ends.

GPS COORDINATES   N 37° 34.272'   W 90° 43.550'

10

Trail of Tears State Park

You'll admire stunning panoramic vistas of the Mississippi River from overlooks in Trail of Tears State Park.

Trail of Tears State Park is a place of both natural beauty and historical significance. The park's name evokes the forced relocation of American Indians from their lands in the Southeast. Called Nunahi-Duna-Dlu-Hilu-I by natives, or "Trail where they cried," their 800-mile trek passed by and through the park. It's estimated that 4,000 people died during the trek to Indian Territory in what is now eastern Oklahoma. In 1987 Congress designated the Trail of Tears a National Historic Trail.

The park's 3,415 acres overlay a maze of ridges and hollows next to the Mississippi River. You'll get a feel for this rugged riverside landscape at the park's visitor center, where a scale model of Trail of Tears shows its topography, including its roads, trails, and campgrounds. The visitor center is a fascinating place—half of it is dedicated to the history of the Trail of Tears, and the rest to the park's natural features. You'll find maps of the trek's two routes, bios of leaders on both the native and settler sides of the forced exodus, and panels with paintings, drawings, and participants' accounts of their travails along the way. The remainder of the center's displays include dioramas of the trees and plants that grow here, geologic history, and mounted displays of the birds and animals you might see at Trail of Tears.

The park's campsites are divided among two campgrounds. If you like being near water, head for the Mississippi River Campground. Located on a flatland next to the river, it has expansive lawn, picnic shelters, and small playground that make it a great place for family camping. Unfortunately, it's the developed campground at Trail of Tears. Because all of its 19 sites have electricity and many have sewer and water service, it's an RV magnet. If you do camp down here, go for sites 13–19. They're electric-only sites on the west side of the loop, nestled against a forested hillside where they'll get afternoon shade, and spaced farther apart than the full-service sites on the loop's east side.

Lake Boutin Campground (open only May–October) is the better place for tent campers. All of its 35 campsites are basic ones. They're scattered along the spine of a Y-shaped ridgeline, with a modern bathhouse and laundry at the junction of the Y. The ridge catches the breeze, and most of the sites along its spine are well shaded. One of the park's trails wanders through the camp, and swimming and fishing in Lake Boutin are only a few hundred yards down the trail. A short walk to the campground

:: Ratings

BEAUTY: ★ ★ ★
PRIVACY: ★ ★ ★ ★
SPACIOUSNESS: ★ ★ ★ ★
QUIET: ★ ★ ★ ★
SECURITY: ★ ★ ★ ★
CLEANLINESS: ★ ★ ★ ★ ★

:: Key Information

ADDRESS: 429 Moccasin Springs Jackson, MO 63755

OPERATED BY: Missouri Department of Natural Resources

CONTACT: Park office, 573-290-5268; mostateparks.com/park/trail-tears-state-park

OPEN: Mississippi River CG: Year-round; Lake Boutin CG: May–Oct.

SITES: 35 basic, 10 electric, 8 full hookup

SITE AMENITIES: Table, fire pit with grate, lantern pole; some with cooking shelters, tent pads

ASSIGNMENT: First come, first served; reservations at 866-ICAMPMO or park's website

REGISTRATION Lake Boutin CG: occupy site, host will collect fee; Mississippi River CG: pay at loop entrance

FACILITIES: Apr.-Oct.: Water, flush toilets, showers, laundry, dump station, beach;

Year-round: Vault toilets, visitor center, playgrounds, picnicking, trails

PARKING: At each site, on pavement

FEE: Apr.-Oct.: $13 basic, $21 electric, $26 full hookup; Nov.-Mar.: $12 basic, $19 electric, $22 full hookup; $8.50 non-refundable reservation fee; $2 discount for seniors or campers with disabilities

ELEVATION: 600' Lake Boutin CG; 380' Mississippi River CG

RESTRICTIONS:

■ **Pets:** On 10-foot leash

■ **Fires:** In fire pits; campers must comply with current firewood advisories

■ **Alcohol:** Allowed in campsites but not in parking lots or on the beach

■ **Vehicles:** Over 25 feet would fit better in Mississippi River CG

■ **Other:** 15-day stay limit; 6-person limit per site; 2-night minimum stay for weekend reservations

entrance leads to one of the park's views of the Mississippi Valley.

Sites 20–30 are located on the entrance road that forms the base of the Y. While they're nice sites, only site 21 has any level tent space. These sites are best suited for camper vans and pickups with camper tops. Beyond the bathhouse the ridge shoulders don't drop off as steeply, so most sites on the west and south arms of the campground have level spots for tents. Sites 51–54 are the best sites on the western arm of the campground. They're on the turnaround loop with views of Lake Boutin. Site 48, a pull-through with lots of space for tents, is another good site on the western arm.

I like the campsites on the southern arm of camp best. Except for sites 39, 40, and 41—they're too close to the restrooms—all

the sites here are good ones. Most are well spaced and shady, and they have level areas for tents. Site 43, located on the outside of a curve in the road, is an excellent site. It's a good distance off the road and has a nice tent pad. My favorite sites are 44 and 45 on the turnaround. They're all by themselves at the end of the road, and site 44 has a secluded tent pad far from the pavement.

Activities at Trail of Tears State Park include swimming, picnicking, and fishing for bass, bluegill, and catfish in Lake Boutin. But for my money, the best feature of the park is its hiking trails. Families will enjoy the half-mile Nature Trail at the visitor center, and campers at Lake Boutin can roam the 2.25-mile Lake Trail right from their campsites. If you camp at the Mississippi River Campground, you'll be near the

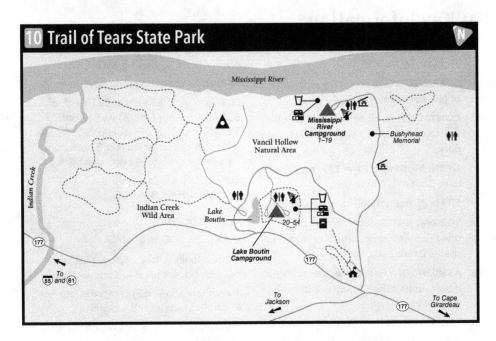

10 Trail of Tears State Park

Mississippi River

Vancil Hollow
Natural Area

Mississippi
River
Campground
1–19

Bushyhead
Memorial

Indian Creek

Indian Creek
Wild Area

Lake
Boutin

20–54

Lake Boutin
Campground

177

To
55 and 61

To
Jackson

177

To Cape
Girardeau

Sheppard Point Trail, a 3-mile hike that alternately climbs to hogback ridges with views of the Mississippi, and then drops steeply to dark, damp riverside hollows.

The best hike in the park, though, is the Peewah Trail. Divided into a yellow loop and a red loop, the Peewah is a 10-mile trail system that can be explored on hikes ranging from 1.25 to 10 miles. The 1.25-mile hike is a scenic jaunt to the Mississippi Overlook and back, and the 10-mile hike is a trek from either of the system's two trailheads, around both loops, and back. Both loops include long stretches in deep hollows and along breezy hogback ridges, but the yellow loop is the prettiest. For 2 miles on its east side you'll parallel the Mississippi, with expansive views across the immense river and into the Illinois hills on its far side. It's good to end your hike on this stretch, where all the scenery give you plenty of excuses to rest your tired feet.

:: Getting There

From I-55 take Exit 105 for Fruitland/Jackson/US 61. From there, signs will lead you to the park. Go northeast 1 mile on US 61 to MO 177. Turn south on MO 177 and follow it 11 miles to the park. Turn left at the first park entrance and drive 0.75 mile east to reach Lake Boutin Campground. To reach the Missouri River Campground, follow MO 177 to the second park entrance, turn left, and follow Moccasin Springs Road 2 miles to the camp.

GPS COORDINATES   N 37° 26.322'   W 89° 28.840'

11

Wallace State Park

Wallace State Park is a peaceful oasis less than an hour's drive from the noise and traffic of the Kansas City metro area.

The 501 acres of wooded hills and bottomlands in Wallace State Park are named for the family that once owned part of this land. The park came into existence in the 1930s through the preservation efforts of the Cameron Sportsman's Club, and its early developmental stages were part of a Works Progress Administration project. It's a beautiful place, featuring forested hills, moist bottomlands, field openings, and a stream with several low waterfalls, all arranged around the park's centerpiece—Lake Allaman, a 6-acre pond with excellent fishing and swimming.

Wallace State Park's campgrounds are divided into five separate camping areas—Campgrounds 1–4 and the special-use area. The best place for tent camping is Campground 1, a 34-site basic campground. Many of its sites have table shelters, and all are incredibly well shaded. Most are private sites separated from their neighbors by brush and woods, so that even those with tight spacing offer good solitude. The best sites are on the northern half of the loop, where better spacing makes for the most seclusion. Sites near the turn of the horseshoe loop are a bit

:: Ratings

BEAUTY: ★ ★ ★ ★
PRIVACY: ★ ★ ★ ★ ★
SPACIOUSNESS: ★ ★ ★ ★
QUIET: ★ ★ ★ ★ ★
SECURITY: ★ ★ ★ ★ ★
CLEANLINESS: ★ ★ ★ ★ ★

close together. Every site has either an inviting grassy tent space or a wood-lined tent pad filled with a soft bed of wood chips.

Sites 1, 3, 7, and 9 are spacious camping spots on the inside of the loop. Each of these has plenty of grassy tent space and good shade, with a comfortable distance from its neighbors. Sites 8, 10, and 11 on the outside of the loop are little wooded alcoves. Their parking spurs reach far from the campground road, and surrounding trees and brush make them second only to the loop's walk-in sites for privacy and seclusion. Sites 12–20 on the end of the horseshoe are good sites, but they're more crowded than the others and somewhat close to the road.

For the most solitude, camp in sites 28–31, the park's four walk-in sites. These are true walk-in sites, not just camping spots a few feet from the road. Site 28 is 250 feet from the parking area, site 29 is 400 feet, site 30 is 750 feet, and site 31 is 850 feet into the woods. It's worth the minor trek to reach these hidden camping spots. Each walk-in site is well shaded, has a soft wood-chip tent pad, and is connected by trails to restrooms and the lake. My favorite is site 30, where larger-than-normal trees shade the campsite.

Campground 2, just south of the basic loop, is another pretty place to camp. All its sites are electric, and it's the place to be if you like open area around your campsite. Sites 41, 44, 45, and 46 are alcove sites in the woods, but Campground 2's remaining

:: Key Information

ADDRESS: 10621 NE MO 121
Cameron, MO 64429

OPERATED BY: Missouri Department
of Natural Resources

CONTACT: Park office, 816-632-3745;
mostateparks.com/park/wallace-state-
park

OPEN: Apr. 15–Oct. 31: 7 a.m.–10 p.m.;
Nov. 1–Apr. 14: 7 a.m.–8 p.m.

SITES: 35 basic, 4 walk-in basic,
42 electric

SITE AMENITIES: Table, fire pit with
grate, lantern pole; some with tent pads
and table shelters

ASSIGNMENT: First come, first served;
reservations at 877-ICAMPMO or park's
website

REGISTRATION: At check station behind
shower house

FACILITIES: Apr. 15–Oct. 31: Flush toilets,
showers, laundry; Year-round: Water,
vault toilets, shelters, amphitheater

PARKING: At each site, on pavement

FEE: Apr. 15–Oct. 31: $13 basic, $21
electric, $23 electric premium; Nov. 1–
Apr. 14: $12 basic, $19 electric, $21 elec-
tric premium; $8.50 nonrefundable
reservation fee; $2 discount for seniors
and campers with disabilities

ELEVATION: 900'

RESTRICTIONS:

■ **Pets:** On 10-foot leash

■ **Fires:** In fire pits; campers must comply with current firewood advisories

■ **Alcohol:** Allowed in campsites but not
in parking lots or in swimming areas

■ **Vehicles:** Electric, up to 70 feet; basic,
up to 50 feet

■ **Other:** 15-day stay limit; 6-person
limit per site; 2-night minimum stay for
weekend reservations

sites are grassy spots with scattered shade trees. It's a pleasant place, with comfortably spaced camping spots along both sides of a horseshoe loop.

Campgrounds 3 and 4 are the southernmost loops at Wallace State Park and are only open April 15–October 31. Campground 3 is another basic campground, a small gravel-road loop with sites 64–68. Because all of its five sites are visible from each other and not very far apart, it's a good place for small groups. There's not much direct shade on this loop, but woods on the west side of all five sites bring shade by midafternoon. Campground 4 is just south of Campground 3. It's similar to Campground 2, with 20 electric sites within a mix of open space and scattered trees. Sites 78, 79, and 80 at the back of the loop, private sites in wooded alcoves, are the best camping spots in Campground 4.

The special-use area is a set of three camps open to youth groups. They're attractive camping spots, each able to hold 30–50 campers, in a private corner of the park with a combination of wide-open space and woods. Contact the park office in advance to reserve one of these group camps.

Wallace State Park is a good destination for families. It has two small playgrounds and an excellent beach on Lake Allaman. Its picnic area has horseshoe pits, a volleyball court, and an open field good for playing ball or tossing a Frisbee.

My favorite feature at Wallace State Park is its trail network. Four trails explore the landscape, and all the park's facilities—campgrounds, lake, and picnic areas—are connected by these trails. In this relatively small park it's an easy walk to the lake from any campground, and by stringing several trails together you can take hikes ranging

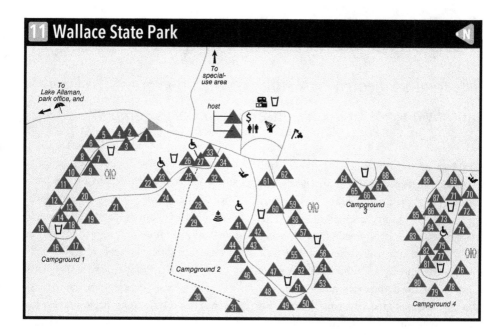

11 Wallace State Park

in length from a few hundred yards to 5 or 6 miles.

The two prettiest hikes in the park are the Rocky Ford and Deer Run Trails. The 0.6-mile Rocky Ford Trail descends from the upper picnic area to several pretty cascades on Deer Creek. It's the hike to take for nice scenery with little effort. For more challenge and a wilder atmosphere, head out on the Deer Run Trail. With hills and some rocky and rooty sections, it's similar to a typical Ozark trail. Cutoffs let you divide this somewhat strenuous hike into loops of 1, 2, or 3 miles, and along its length you'll enjoy fields, forests, creeks, and ponds.

:: Getting There

From Exit 48 on I-35, go a half mile south on US 69 to MO 121. Go east on MO 121 and follow it 1.5 miles into the park. The turnoff to the campgrounds is on the left a quarter mile down the park road, just before you reach Lake Allaman.

GPS COORDINATES   N 39° 39.336'   W 94° 12.647'

12

Washington State Park

The weather-beaten rock stairs on the 1,000 Steps Trail were built by a 1930s Civilian Conservation Corps company.

On top of the pretty hills, hollows, and streams you expect to find in the Ozark landscapes, Washington State Park is also rich in both history and prehistory. The rustic cabins, lodge, headquarters, overlook shelters, and rough-hewn stone trail steps were built by a Civilian Conservation Corps company in the 1930s, and long before the CCC artisans made their mark here, the park's prehistoric inhabitants carved two-thirds of Missouri's known petroglyphs on rock outcrops in the park's 1,875 acres. While these are the features that landed Washington State Park on the National Register of Historic Places, the park's natural beauty is pretty good too. Dolomite bluffs tower over a picnic ground nestled in a bend of the Big River, and winding trails lead to spectacular overlooks of the river valley.

Washington State Park is a great place for families. There's an Olympic-size swimming pool not far from the campground, and those who like their water a little wilder can take a dip in the Big River at the river access in the picnic area. Anglers fish for bass, bluegill, and catfish, and you can rent canoes,

rafts, or tubes at the Thunderbird Lodge to explore the river above and below the park. Visits to the petroglyph panels are educational for folks of any age, and if someone in your family or group isn't into camping, the park has nice cabins for rent.

For me, the campground's the place. The road forks as you enter the camp, with electric sites on the right, basic sites on the left, and the bathhouse, amphitheater, and a small playground at the junction. The electric sites are nice: they're shady and fairly well spaced, with lots of grass around many of the sites. Sites on the outside of the road on this L-shaped loop are the farthest apart, and sites 19 and 20 at the very back are the most private sites. They're also close to the Opossum Trail, which passes northeast of the loop. Site 13 is a family site.

The basic sites are scattered along a ridge that runs northwest from the campground entrance. Some are more level than others, but all have level spaces for tents. The first sites along the ridge, sites 26–31 and 46–51, offer the best spacing. The closer you get to the end of the ridge, the closer the sites are to each other. This makes sites 32–44, which are closed November–March, the least attractive to those wishing for privacy. Hikers might prefer those at the end of the campground drive because they're close to a spur leading to the Rockywood Trail. Whichever end of the camp you choose, most sites on the basic side of the campground are good

:: Ratings

BEAUTY: ★ ★ ★ ★
PRIVACY: ★ ★ ★
SPACIOUSNESS: ★ ★ ★ ★
QUIET: ★ ★ ★ ★ ★
SECURITY: ★ ★ ★ ★ ★
CLEANLINESS: ★ ★ ★ ★ ★

:: Key Information

ADDRESS: 13041 MO 104
DeSoto, MO 63020

OPERATED BY: Missouri Department
of Natural Resources

CONTACT: Park office, 636-586-5768;
Thunderbird Lodge, 636-586-2995;
mostateparks.com/park/washington-
state-park

OPEN: Year-round, sunrise–sunset

SITES: 26 basic, 24 electric

SITE AMENITIES: Table, fire grate,
lantern pole

ASSIGNMENT: First come, first served;
reservations at 877-ICAMPMO or park's
website

REGISTRATION Pay campground host at
site 1 or at park office

FACILITIES: Apr.–Oct.: Water, showers,
pool; Year-round: Picnic shelters, store,
cabins, trails, canoe rentals

PARKING: At each site

FEE: Apr.–Oct.: $13 basic, $21 electric,
$36 family electric; Nov.–Mar.: $12
basic, $19 electric, $32 family electric;
$8.50 nonrefundable reservation fee; $2
discount for seniors and campers with
disabilities

ELEVATION: 850'

RESTRICTIONS:

■ **Pets:** On 10-foot leash

■ **Fires:** In fire pits; campers must comply with current firewood advisories

■ **Alcohol:** Allowed in campsites and
picnic areas but not in parking lots or on
beaches

■ **Vehicles:** Electric sites, up to 80 feet;
basic, 20–40 feet

■ **Other:** 15-day stay limit; 6-person
limit per site; 2-night minimum stay for
weekend reservations

ones, and because they are on a dead-end road, they're quiet places.

Whether you're going canoeing or hiking, the Thunderbird Lodge is the place to start. The park's three trails fan out from the lodge, and you can rent canoes, rafts, or tubes there. Floats of 3 or 7 miles are available, with varying departure times. Thunderbird Lodge is an attraction in itself with its impressive CCC stone-and-log construction. It takes its name from one of the park's most interesting petroglyphs and is built directly over a creek. You can stand on the lodge's veranda and watch the stream flow beneath the structure and tumble into the Big River a few yards away.

The 1.5-mile 1,000 Steps Trail showcases more of the CCC's impressive construction accomplishments. Heading east from the Thunderbird Lodge, it climbs onto the bluff

south of the picnic area and travels over worn stone stairs that were manhandled into place by those 1930s stonemasons. They must have been tough—I sure wouldn't want to wrestle with those stones in Missouri's summer heat and humidity. The trail winds over cliffs and rock outcrops on its way to a stone-and-log overlook shelter with a stupendous view of the Big River Valley.

The 2.5-mile Opossum Trail goes south from Thunderbird Lodge, traveling along the creek that flows under the lodge. It follows the stream almost to its headwaters before breaking north and climbing up to the swimming pool, wandering past the campground and cabin area, and then bursting out of the forest at a scenic overlook from a sheer cliff high above the Big River. From there, the trail descends quickly back to the lodge, following the cliff edge for most of the way.

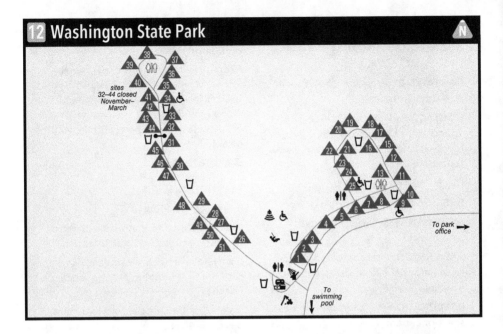

The 7-mile Rockywood Trail is the longest and wildest hike in the park. It's a wonderful all-day hike and has a backpack camp near a spring for those who want to stay out there a little longer. It shares treadway with the best parts of the Opossum and 1,000 Steps Trails, so it shows you all the good scenery in Washington State Park in one long hike. Along its length you'll pass spectacular overlooks, wander through deep hollows, meander through grassy glades, and tramp along breezy ridges. It also passes the petroglyph area, where interpretive displays describe these ancient American Indian works of art and speculate on their meaning.

:: Getting There

Drive 9 miles south from DeSoto on MO 21 to MO 104, which is the road through Washington State Park. Turn right on MO 104 and follow it 2.5 miles to the campground on the right side of the road.

GPS COORDINATES N 38° 5.126' W 90° 41.696'

13

Weston Bend State Park

Admire sweeping vistas from the Missouri River overlooks.

Named for a nearby town on a sweeping curve in the Missouri River, Weston Bend State Park is a place of beauty and pioneer history. American Indians once roamed the park's hills, and Lewis and Clark passed through on their trek to the Pacific in July of 1804. The park is located in Missouri's Loess Hills, a range of hills reaching from just north of Kansas City all the way to Iowa. Loess, fine sediment left behind when glaciers retreated, was blown into mounds by the Midwest's strong winds, and then eroded by streams into the landscape seen today in Weston Bend State Park—forested hills, deep ravines, and small patches of prairie grassland.

The rich loess soil around Weston Bend gave rise to thriving hemp and tobacco farms. For a short time in the mid-1800s their production made nearby Weston the second-largest port on the Missouri River, second only to St. Louis. Founded in 1837 in a natural harbor on the Missouri, Weston grew to 5,000 residents by the 1850s and was the largest hemp port in the world. In 1858 the McCormick Distillery opened, and it continues making firewater to this day. The land around Weston Bend still

:: Ratings

BEAUTY: ★ ★ ★
PRIVACY: ★ ★ ★
SPACIOUSNESS: ★ ★ ★
QUIET: ★ ★ ★ ★
SECURITY: ★ ★ ★ ★ ★
CLEANLINESS: ★ ★ ★ ★ ★

produces tobacco, and five old tobacco barns still stand in the park. One of these has been converted into a shelter and another into an interpretive display.

You can explore the area's beauty and history from the park's pleasant campground. Unfortunately, most of Weston's campsites were electrified in the last few years, but because the park and its namesake town are such interesting places, I've included it anyway. Weston's 35 sites are laid out in a loop, with sites in its western half on a low hilltop and its eastern sites on a wooded flat. Site 1, a family site, and site 3 are basic camping spots just east of the loop entrance with plenty of shade and good spacing. Site 4 is an electric site, but it's a nice private spot surrounded by trees and well shaded. Sites 5–25 are all electric sites that are a bit close together on the northeast side of the loop. They're a little exposed, but are good for off-season camping when a little sunshine is welcome.

After site 25, the campground road crosses a creek, and then comes to site 26, my favorite camping spot at Weston Bend. Trees surround and shade it, and it's a long way from any other site. Water is available just down the road, and a path leads straight across the loop to the bathhouse. It's a great site! Just beyond it the road climbs a short way, and then curves past sites 27–37, the loop's hilltop campsites. These have all recently been wired for 50-amp electric service but still offer many good places for tenting. Site 27 is a good

:: Key Information

ADDRESS: 16600 MO 45 North
Weston, MO 64098-0115

OPERATED BY: Missouri Department
of Natural Resources

CONTACT: Park office, 816-640-5443;
mostateparks.com/park/weston-bend-
state-park

OPEN: Apr. 15–Oct. 31: 7 a.m.–10 p.m.;
Nov. 1–Apr. 14: 7 a.m.–6 p.m.

SITES: 2 basic, 1 basic family, 22 electric,
9 premium electric, 1 family premium
electric

SITE AMENITIES: Table, fire pit with
grate, lantern pole

ASSIGNMENT: First come, first served;
reservations at 888-ICAMPMO or park's
website

REGISTRATION Self-pay station at restrooms near loop entrance

FACILITIES: Water, showers, laundry,
pavilion, dump station, trails, picnic sites

PARKING: At each site, on pavement

FEE: Apr. 15.–Oct. 31: $13 basic, $26
family basic, $21 electric, $23 premium
electric, $46 family premium electric;
Nov. 1–Apr. 14: $12 basic, $24 basic
family, $19 electric, $21 premium electric, $42 family premium electric; $8.50
nonrefundable reservation fee; $2
discount for seniors and campers
with disabilities

ELEVATION: 900'

RESTRICTIONS:

■ **Pets:** On 10-foot leash

■ **Fires:** In fire pits; campers must comply with current firewood advisories

■ **Alcohol:** Allowed in campsites but not
in parking lots and public areas

■ **Vehicles:** Up to 40 feet

■ **Other:** 15-day stay limit; 6-person
limit per site; 2-night minimum stay for
weekend reservations Apr. 15–Oct. 31

spot, well spaced from its neighbors. Site 30 has little shade, but sites 29 and 31, though placed close together, are nice spots shaded by a big tree. My favorite sites on this hill-top are 32, 33, 34, and 37. Though they're not very spacious, they're shady sites on the outside of the loop, tucked into semi-private nooks in the brush with nothing but woods behind them.

There's plenty to do while camping in Weston Bend, both inside and outside of the park. Weston Bend has eight trails to explore. One of these is the hiking-biking path, a 2.7-mile asphalt trail that explores the loess hills in the park center. The 0.3-mile Missouri River Trail meanders through the bottomlands to a beautiful streamside view of the wide, muddy river. The 0.2-mile Bear Creek Trail splits from the Missouri

River Trail and leads to the old channel left by the river when it changed course in 1858, leaving Weston high and dry. The 0.7-mile Campground Trail is an easy hike that begins across from the restroom, and the 3.25-mile Weston Bluffs Trail is a hiking-biking route along the park's western boundary that connects the towns of Weston and Beverly. Its northern half is paved, making for an easy bike ride or walk from the park to Weston's quaint downtown.

Weston Bend's prettiest hikes are the 2-mile out-and-back North Ridge Trail and a 2.5-mile loop using segments of the Harpst, West Ridge, and Paved Bicycle Trails. The North Ridge follows an old road to loess bluffs with a nice vista of the river valley. The Harpst–West Ridge–Paved Bicycle Trail loop wanders through all the varied landscapes

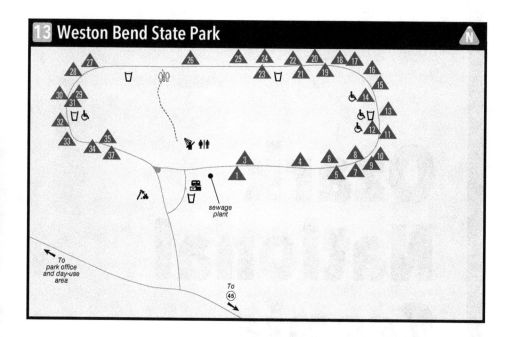

13 Weston Bend State Park

on display at Weston Bend, including several wonderful overlooks. At the trailhead there's a spectacular view across the river valley to Leavenworth on the Kansas side.

The displays at the Tobacco Barn are worth checking out. They explain the tobacco production process and describe tobacco's effect on Weston and the surrounding counties. Several interpretive panels tell the story of American Indian activities around Weston Bend, while others focus on the development of the town of Weston.

When you get hungry, thirsty, or get the urge to shop in a quaint 1850s setting, drive 3 miles northwest to the village of Weston. Its downtown is a step back to the town's days as a thriving river port. Weston features numerous restaurants, craft stores, antiques shops, coffee shops, and a traditional hardware store in its walker-friendly downtown. If you have a hankering for an adult beverage, you'll find an Irish brewpub in the vaults of an 1840s brewery, whiskey sampling and sales at the McCormick Distillery's shop, and a winery with a tasting room and a wine garden where you can enjoy your purchases with bread, cheese, and summer sausage. For those really hot days, a traditional soda fountain serves cold treats made the old-fashioned way.

:: Getting There

From I-29 take Exit 20 for MO 273 North/Tracy/Weston. Go west 0.2 mile to MO 273, and then continue straight ahead on MO 273 for 4.5 miles to MO 45. Go left on MO 45 for 0.5 mile to the park entrance. Turn right into the park and go 0.5 mile to the campground on the right side of the park road.

GPS COORDINATES   N 39° 23.642'   W 94° 52.263'

Ozark National Scenic Riverways

14

Alley Spring

Historic Alley Mill, perched on a beautiful blue-green spring pool, is all that remains of a once-thriving community on the Jacks Fork River.

Alley Spring may be a big campground, but it's a wonderful place to camp in the Ozark National Scenic Riverways. It's not merely a pretty place on the Jacks Fork River, but a historical one as well. The Alley community once thrived in this river bottom, anchored by the Alley Mill, which still stands next to the deep, clear pool of Alley Spring. When you're not on the river, you can hike a trail around the millpond or explore the old mill on one of the organized tours offered during the summer months.

The campground at Alley is large, but don't let campsite numbers as high as 925 fool you—it doesn't have that many sites. It's the campground numbering system that results in big numbers. The campground is laid out in a series of loops containing 20–30 sites each. The first loop contains sites 101–126, the second 202–220, and so on, all the way up to 901–925. There are eight total loops, and a set of walk-in campsites numbered 701–720. Restrooms and water are liberally scattered throughout the four

:: Ratings

BEAUTY: ★ ★ ★ ★ ★
PRIVACY: ★ ★ ★
SPACIOUSNESS: ★ ★ ★
QUIET: ★ ★ ★
SECURITY: ★ ★ ★ ★ ★
CLEANLINESS: ★ ★ ★ ★ ★

loops on the north side of the campground, and each of the four south loops has its own restroom and water supply.

The loops north of the main campground are closest to the river and have the most shade. I'm amazed at the lush grass is on these loops. In most campgrounds with good shade, the grass is anemic. Not so here—Alley has one of the best combinations of grass and shade I've ever seen. Loop 101–126 is closest to the action at Alley Spring. It's near the ranger station, river access, and the pedestrian bridge that goes over Jacks Fork to Alley Mill. All of the sites here are fine places to pitch a tent, but I especially like sites 117–121, which are walk-ins behind the ranger station. They are spacious and shaded, and they have plenty of open lawn around them. Loop 201–220 is a twin to 101–126, and the two share restrooms, showers, and water supply.

The remaining two northside loops, 301–320 and 501–521, are separate from each other. Sites there are a little farther apart, and each loop has its own restroom and bathhouse. They have the same excellent shade and grass as the first two loops, with more space and less activity. My favorite sites on these two loops are 303, 316, and 508, because they sit amid an open grassy area. Walk-ins 701–725 are west of the 500 loop and are scattered under shade trees. Located in the far end of the campground,

:: Key Information

ADDRESS: 404 Watercress Dr., P.O. Box 490, Van Buren, MO 63965

OPERATED BY: National Park Service

CONTACT: 573-323-4236; nps.gov/ozar

OPEN: Year-round

SITES: 143 individual, 19 walk-in, 3 group

SITE AMENITIES: Table, fire pit with grate, lantern pole, parking pad; some sites have electricity and water

ASSIGNMENT: First come, first served; reservations (required for group sites) available at 877-444-6777 or recreation.gov

REGISTRATION: Self-pay at campground entrance

FACILITIES: Apr. 16–Oct. 14: Water, flush toilets, showers, store; Year-round: Historic sites, river access, canoe rental, trails

PARKING: At each site, on pavement

FEE: Apr. 16–Oct. 14: $14 individual, $17 electric/water, $30 cluster, $100 group; Oct. 15–Apr. 15: free

ELEVATION: 670'

RESTRICTIONS:

■ **Pets:** On 6-foot leash

■ **Fires:** In fire pits; burn only firewood gathered or purchased locally

■ **Alcohol:** Allowed, subject to local ordinances

■ **Vehicles:** Up to 30 feet

■ **Other:** 14-day stay limit; no glass containers in caves or within 50 feet of river; 6-person, 2-tent limit per site; no swimming in Alley Spring or creek; quiet hours 10 p.m.–6 a.m.

these are among the most peaceful sites at Alley Spring.

The four loops to the south of the main camp road are more open than those near the river and offer a mix of shady and sunny sites. Woods ring the outside of the loops, with sites tucked into the trees, and groves of trees shade many sites on the inside of each circle. Loop 401–429 contains cluster sites, which have parking for two cars and space for 7–20 people. You'll need to get permission from a ranger before using these. Loop 601–628 has the sites with electric and water hookups, but few are well shaded. Loop 801–830 is very nice, with many shady sites on both the inside and outside of the loop road. It's close to the camp amphitheater, so expect some evening foot traffic when there's an interpretive talk.

Of the four southside loops, 901–925 is my favorite. It's at the back of the camp where it's likely to be quiet, and it has the most shaded sites. If it's cool, I can pick an open, sunny site, and there's even a little room to toss a Frisbee around without hitting other campers. It feels like a little camp that is all its own—perfect if you like lots of privacy like I do.

Alley is a great place to hang out—everyone knows about the canoeing here. You can rent canoes at the store across from the entrance, as well as most things you'll need for your float or campout. You have a nice choice of floats at Alley. One laid-back trip is the easy 7-mile float to Eminence. More committed paddlers can enjoy the wilder 24-mile float from MO 17 to Alley Spring. That adventure floats past Meeting House Cave, the gaping maw of Jam Up Cave, and beneath several towering bluffs—a two- or three-day float that will have you looking forward to the hot showers at Alley.

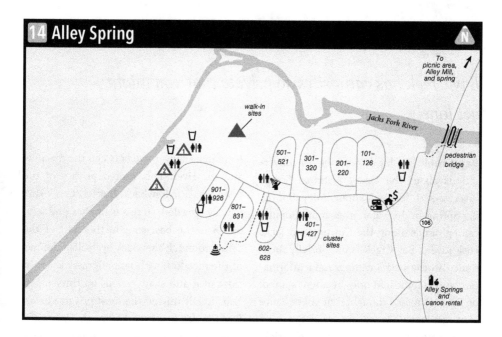

When you tire of the river, hike the pedestrian bridge to the historic area across Jacks Fork from camp. The old Story's Creek School, a one-room schoolhouse moved to Alley in 1971, is an interesting attraction, but the biggest draw is the old mill. Built in the 1890s, Alley Mill is a fascinating place, with tours available June–August. A 0.3-mile trail wanders around the spring's pool, and the 1.5-mile Alley Overlook Trail climbs the bluff above the mill. Once you top the bluff, you'll have a dizzying view straight down into the spring pond and a panorama of smoky hills to the south. Fall is an especially magical time to visit Alley Spring—crimson and yellow leaves float in the blue-green waters of the millpond, and bright autumn colors splash the hillsides.

For even better views of the countryside, drive 5 miles west on MO 106 to its junction with MO D. There you'll find the Flat Rock Tower, an old fire lookout with expansive views over miles and miles of Ozark hills. You'll be huffing and puffing when you get to the top, but the scenery is worth the climb.

:: Getting There

Drive 5 miles west from Eminence on MO 106 to Alley Spring. The campground entrance will be on your left just before you cross Jacks Fork. Alley Mill and the picnic area are across the river.

GPS COORDINATES N 37° 8.656' W 91° 26.636'

15

Bay Creek

Bay Creek has campsites so private that you might get lonely.

Bay Creek is a bit of a secret. In conversations about the Ozark National Scenic Riverways, I learned about Alley Spring, Big Spring, and several other more popular campgrounds along the Current and Jacks Fork Rivers. Bay Creek is only briefly mentioned in the park's campground information and is indicated only by a tent symbol on the park map. I thought it might be a nice spot—and it sure is.

Located where tiny Bay Creek trickles into Jacks Fork River, this backwoods hideaway doesn't have all the amenities of the large campground at nearby Alley Spring, but it also doesn't have the crowds. It does have swimming, wading, fishing, a huge bluff towering over the river, old doubletrack roads for hiking and mountain biking, and campsites so private that you might get lonely. If you do want some company or a shower, Alley Spring is only a few miles away.

The main camp loop is on the right as you enter Bay Creek. Sites 1–4 are in a grassy meadow with shady edges, and sites 5 and 6 are in a shady grove between the meadow and the river. The limited privacy of the open area is a drawback. But Bay Creek isn't usually crowded, so this is rarely a problem. Site 4 is the best spot in this part of the campground. It's set back by itself at the end of the meadow, with lots of grassy space in front of it and shady woods on three sides. You already missed the most private site on Bay Creek's north end, though. A narrow gravel road that breaks left off the entrance drive just north of the main loop leads to an unnumbered roomy campsite perched right on the river's edge. It's not well shaded but is very secluded.

For real privacy, splash through the Bay Creek ford and drive the skinny and forbidding road up the hill beyond. It climbs onto a pretty bench about 20 feet above the river and follows it for almost 2 miles. About a half mile past the main campground on your left, you'll see site 7 nestled under shade trees next to the river. It's the best site in Bay Creek. A quarter mile beyond is a vault toilet. Just past the vault toilet you'll find site 8 on the right. It's another very private site, but it isn't well shaded. Another mile upriver, the road ends near sites 9 and 10 next to Jacks Fork River. Site 9 is a little rough, but site 10 is a wonderful hideaway next to a soothing riffle on Jacks Fork. All four sites on this road are wonderfully secluded. From the last two sites it's an easy hike along gravel bars to Bee Bluff just upstream.

:: Ratings

BEAUTY: ★ ★ ★ ★
PRIVACY: ★ ★ ★ ★ ★
SPACIOUSNESS: ★ ★ ★ ★ ★
QUIET: ★ ★ ★ ★ ★
SECURITY: ★ ★ ★ ★
CLEANLINESS: ★ ★ ★ ★

:: Key Information

ADDRESS: 404 Watercress Dr., P.O. Box 490, Van Buren, MO 63965

OPERATED BY: National Park Service

CONTACT: 573-323-4236; nps.gov/ozar

OPEN: Year-round

SITES: 11

SITE AMENITIES: Table, fire pit with grate, trash can, grill, lantern pole

ASSIGNMENT: First come, first served

REGISTRATION: Self-registration at pay station

FACILITIES: Vault toilets, river access

PARKING: At each site

FEE: Apr. 16–Oct. 14: $5; Oct. 15– Apr. 15: free

ELEVATION: 720'

RESTRICTIONS:

▓ **Pets:** On 6-foot leash

▓ **Fires:** In fire pits, rings, or pans; burn only firewood gathered or purchased locally

▓ **Alcohol:** Allowed, subject to local ordinances

▓ **Vehicles:** Up to 20 feet

▓ **Other:** 14-day stay limit; no glass containers in caves or within 50 feet of river; 6-person, 2-vehicle limit per site; quiet hours 10 p.m.–6 a.m.

Between the last two sites a road past the toilet climbs steeply to the north, forking about 100 feet up the hill. If your car can climb this road, take the left fork for a quarter mile. There you'll find an unofficial campsite—just a fire ring and a parking spot—at the base of massive Bee Bluff towering over the river. From this site you can explore a nice gravel bar in the river below the tall bluff. The right fork of this road climbs gradually to the hills north of the river. Grab your boots or bike and head up this road to explore the forests along the Ozark National Scenic Riverways.

The road along the river makes Bay Creek an ideal place for tubing. Fend off summer heat by repeatedly hiking upriver and tubing the Jacks Fork back to camp. Upstream from Bay Creek is one of the most beautiful and remote parts of the Jacks Fork. An 18-mile float from MO 17 down to the campground goes past Jam Up Cave, Meeting House Cave, Ebb and Flow Spring, and several impressive bluffs. On the way over to the put-in, stop at the intersection of MO 106 and MO D and climb the Flat Rock Lookout Tower for expansive vistas from a 1,244-foot elevation.

For a taste of Missouri history and folkways, drive 5 miles east to Alley Mill and Spring. Built in 1894, the mill rises three stories above a blue-green spring that gushes 81 million clear, cool gallons every day. The first two floors of this picturesque mill are open daily, Memorial Day–Labor Day. A 0.3-mile path goes around the spring pool and crosses a stream roaring through the old millrace. The 1.5-mile Overlook Trail climbs to the bluff 100 feet above the mill complex. An interpretive display at the overlook describes life in the community that once occupied the lowlands between the spring and the river.

The old Story's Creek School sits on the west side of the spring branch below Alley Mill. The Alley community had a school in the old days, but it's long gone. Story's Creek School was moved to Alley Spring in 1971 from another location 4 miles away and is open on weekends Memorial Day– Labor Day.

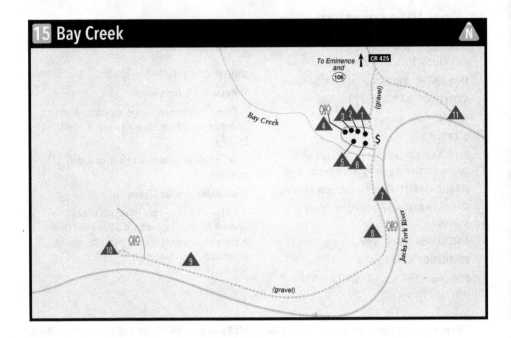

:: Getting There

Drive 9.5 miles west from Eminence on MO 106 to Shannon County Road 106/425, where a sign directs you to Bay Creek. Turn left and follow this gravel county road 2.3 miles to Bay Creek. It's a rough road, but if my Mazda 626 can make it, your vehicle probably can too. To help you find Bay Creek, GPS coordinates are for the campground itself, not the turnoff on MO 106.

GPS COORDINATES   N 37° 7.280'   W 91° 30.287'

16

Big Spring

Big Spring, one of Missouri's first state parks, features charming Civilian Conservation Corps stonework in its cabins, lodge, and entrance station.

Big Spring's history as a public recreation area dates to 1924, when it became one of Missouri's first state parks. In 1969 Missouri donated this jewel to the National Park Service to be part of the newly established Ozark National Scenic Riverways. Now thousands of visitors come to this lovely area on the lower Current River to enjoy canoeing, hiking, scenic drives, dinner at the park's rustic Civilian Conservation Corps–era lodge, and, of course, camping next to the river in Big Spring's expansive campground. For those outdoor enthusiasts who prefer a little decadence with their outdoor fun, 14 comfortable cabins await.

Until spring of 2013, Big Spring Campground was open year-round. Due to the budget sequester in March of that year, the camp's season was reduced to Memorial Day weekend–Labor Day. Ranger talks and other activities on the riverways were reduced, and the Ozark Heritage Day event described later was canceled. The budget issues may have been resolved by the time

you wish to camp at Big Spring, resulting in a longer season and restoration of the area's events. Check the Ozark Riverways website before planning your trip, and you'll know if you can head for Big Spring during Missouri's wonderful spring and fall camping seasons.

Big Spring's individual campsites are laid out in six loops at the far northeast end of the recreation area. The 100 and 200 loops, with sites 101–124 and 202–229, respectively, offer the best camping at Big Spring. Sites in the 100 loop are all basic, while the 200s are electric sites. They're on a spur road to your right as you enter camp. These two loops are better shaded than the others and are closest to the river. Sites on the outside of the loop are more spacious, private, and shady than those in the center. Campsite 114 is my favorite—it's a shady and secluded camping spot near the stairs to the river.

The remaining four loops lie in a meadow a bit farther north on the campground road. The two loops containing sites 301–319 and 401–421 are somewhat tightly spaced and lack good shade, but they do offer level expanses of lush grass for your tent. The loop with sites 501–518 is laid out like the previous two, but shade is somewhat better there. The 600 loop, sites 601–620, offers more spacious and shaded camping than the other four meadow loops. Campsites 605 and 606 at the back of the loop are

:: Ratings

BEAUTY: ★ ★ ★ ★ ★

PRIVACY: ★ ★

SPACIOUSNESS: ★ ★ ★ ★

QUIET: ★ ★ ★ ★

SECURITY: ★ ★ ★ ★ ★

CLEANLINESS: ★ ★ ★ ★ ★

:: Key Information

ADDRESS: 404 Watercress Dr., P.O. Box 490, Van Buren, MO 63965

OPERATED BY: National Park Service

CONTACT: 573-323-4236; nps.gov/ozar; bigspringlodgeandcabins.com (concessionaire)

OPEN: Memorial Day weekend–Labor Day; longer season likely in future years

SITES: 102 basic, 28 electric, 3 group

SITE AMENITIES: Table, lantern pole, fire pit with grate

ASSIGNMENT: First come, first served; reservations available at 877-444-6777 or at recreation.gov

REGISTRATION: At pay station at campground entrance

FACILITIES: Water, restrooms, showers, pavilion, river access, trails, dining lodge, cabins

PARKING: At each site

FEE: Apr. 16–Oct. 14: $14 basic, $17 electric, $100 group, $50 Chubb Hollow group site; Oct. 15–Apr. 15: free (if open)

ELEVATION: 455'

RESTRICTIONS:

■ **Pets:** On 6-foot leash

■ **Fires:** In fire pits; burn only firewood gathered or purchased locally

■ **Alcohol:** Allowed, subject to local ordinances

■ **Vehicles:** Up to 50 feet

■ **Other:** 14-day stay limit; no glass containers in caves or within 50 feet of river; 6-person, 2-vehicle limit per site; quiet hours 10 p.m.–6 a.m.

the best campsites here. All sites are close to restrooms and water.

On the way to camp you passed by all the amenities the recreation area has to offer. Big Spring, the campground's namesake feature, is the star attraction. It's a stunning spot, and the facts behind it are equally impressive. It gushes an average of 286 million gallons a day from beneath a towering cliff, forming the Current's second-largest tributary with its 1,000-foot spring branch flowing to the river. It's one of the world's 10 largest springs, and dye tracings indicate that it draws water from up to 40 miles away. The seeping rainwater welling up at Big Spring is slightly acidic, dissolving the underlying limestone and carrying 173 tons of sediment each day from deep in the earth. These fine limestone particles give the water its aquamarine tinge as it rushes down to the Current River.

North of the spring is the Depression Farm, a few rustic buildings that resemble structures the early Current River pioneers might have built in the early 1900s. This is the site for Ozark Heritage Day, an annual event featuring music, storytellers, and craft demonstrations showcasing skills necessary to wrest a living from these rugged hills and hollows. Usually held in June, this event was canceled in 2013 due to the budget sequester, but the park hopes to revive it in future years.

The park's cabin and lodge are as beautiful as they are historic. From 1933 to 1937 companies 734, 1710, and 1740 of the Civilian Conservation Corps lived and worked at Big Spring. In addition to the cabins and lodge, "The C's" built trails, put up a fire tower, cleared brush to prevent forest fires, and constructed dikes to keep the river out of Big Spring. A fascinating interpretive display near the dining lodge describes the

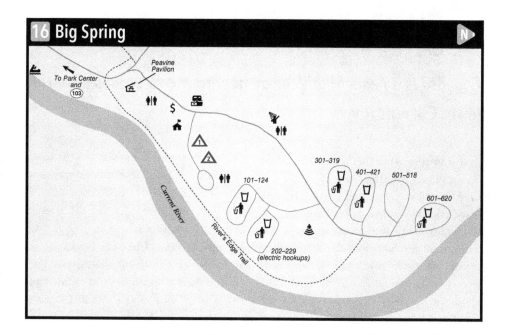

work and daily life of these young men during their time in camp at Big Spring.

With an extensive trail system linking all the attractions at Big Spring, hiking is the perfect way to leisurely explore everything that's here. The River's Edge Trail begins in the campground. You can hike it to the Slough Trail, follow the Slough Trail to Big Spring, and then follow the Spring Branch Trail to the dining lodge on an easy hike of about 2.5 miles one-way. You can also combine the wheelchair-accessible Slough Trail with the rugged Stone Ridge Trail for a 2.5-mile loop exploring an abandoned river channel through wetlands and canebrakes, which then ascends over stone steps hewed by the CCC to rugged bluffs overlooking Big Spring.

At 4 miles, the Chubb Hollow Trail is the longest ramble at Big Spring. Starting from the dining lodge parking lot, it travels a short way along the base of a riverside bluff, climbs to vistas of the Current and Big Spring, ascends to the Big Spring Fire Tower, and explores the Big Spring Pines State Natural Area, home to a pine-oak forest. On its way back to the dining lodge, it passes through the old CCC encampment, and then returns to civilization near the cabins built by the young men who once lived in the now-forested camp site. Other trails connecting to the Chubb Hollow Trail extend even farther into the riverways scenic landscape. The Trails Illustrated map *Ozark National Scenic Riverways* is a great help in finding your way along Big Spring's trail system.

:: Getting There

From Van Buren drive west across the Current River on US 60 to MO 103, and then turn south and follow MO 103 4 miles to Big Spring.

GPS COORDINATES   N 36° 57.667'   W 90° 59.151'

17

Logyard

Logyard is a peaceful hideaway next to the clear waters of the lower Current River.

In the southern part of the Ozark National Scenic Riverways, the Current is a wide, deep, and clear stream, and Logyard is a fine place to enjoy boating, fishing, canoeing, or swimming in this beautiful river. Logyard is a tiny primitive campground with only vault toilets and water, so it's not heavily used. Known and accessed mostly by locals, this laid-back hideaway is a rustic escape for those who prefer avoiding more developed campgrounds like Round Spring, Two Rivers, or Alley Spring.

Logyard has seven official sites, and dispersed camping is allowed on Logyard Bar. The seven regular sites are evenly spaced around a grassy, open area shaded by hardwoods. Though all sites are visible from each other, they're spaced just far enough to give you the personal space you need. All sites are shaded and have plenty of space around them for two tents. There are no roads to the sites—only some gravel parking spaces on the road passing through camp—but if it hasn't rained recently, you can park on the grass next to your site.

:: Ratings

BEAUTY: ★ ★ ★ ★
PRIVACY: ★ ★ ★
SPACIOUSNESS: ★ ★ ★ ★ ★
QUIET: ★ ★ ★ ★ ★
SECURITY: ★ ★ ★ ★
CLEANLINESS: ★ ★ ★

The Current River is 100 yards to the south of camp, separated from the campground by a band of riverside trees.

The best place to enjoy the river at Logyard is another half mile upriver from the campground. There the road ends on an expansive gravel bar that slopes gently into the Current River, with a low bluff rising from its opposite side. The gravel beach is the perfect place to swim, sunbathe, or beach your canoe or boat. You can pitch your tent on Logyard Bar too, and there's one semiprivate camping spot on a shaded knoll overlooking the river.

The official river access at Logyard is just east of the T-intersection at the end of MO HH. The gravel road continues downriver beyond the access, and if you feel a little adventurous, you should follow it on downstream. It is an adventure because the road soon turns rough, and 0.75 mile east of the T-intersection it drops into a wash and follows it a few yards south to the Current River. This is a pretty little spot along the river that you'll probably have all to yourself. Be careful in the wash—if there has been water there lately, you might get stuck. If in doubt, visit this spot by hiking the road from the river access. This little place is a great tubing destination. You could float down from the gravel beach and walk back to camp on the road.

Other than fishing, canoeing, boating, and swimming, Logyard doesn't offer lots

:: Key Information

ADDRESS: 404 Watercress Dr., P.O. Box 490, Van Buren, MO 63965

OPERATED BY: National Park Service

CONTACT: 573-323-4236; nps.gov/ozar

OPEN: Year-round

SITES: 7; open camping allowed on Logyard gravel bar

SITE AMENITIES: Table, fire pit with grate, lantern pole; more limited amenities on Logyard Bar

ASSIGNMENT: First come, first served

REGISTRATION: Self-pay at loop entrance

FACILITIES: Apr. 16–Oct. 14: Water; Year-round: Vault toilets, river access

PARKING: At each site

FEE: Apr. 16–Oct. 14: $5; Oct. 15–Apr. 15: free

ELEVATION: 650'

RESTRICTIONS:

■ **Pets:** On 6-foot leash

■ **Fires:** In fire pits; burn only firewood gathered or purchased locally

■ **Alcohol:** Allowed, subject to local ordinances

■ **Vehicles:** Up to 30 feet

■ **Other:** 14-day stay limit; no glass containers in caves or within 50 feet of river; 6-person, 2-tent limit per site; quiet hours 10 p.m.–6 a.m.

of activities—no trails pass by camp, and no caves, overlooks, or other special natural features grace its environs. It's just a nice get-away-from-it-all hangout in the woods, where you'll usually share the campground with only a few other people. If you're willing to explore, though, you're only a short drive to many historic sites in the Ozark National Scenic Riverways.

The closest of these is Blue Spring, about 10 miles upriver from Logyard near the Powder Mill Campground. You can drive to the spring on a gravel road off MO 106, or hike to this gem on a 1-mile trail from Powder Mill. The easy jaunt follows the Current River from Powder Mill to the spring, with the stream at your side all the way. Once at the spring, you'll be amazed at how gorgeous it is—90 million gallons of clear blue water gush daily from a 300-foot-deep cavern, with bubbles wavering upward from its depths. The creek flowing from Blue Spring to the Current, held at a constant temperature year-round by the water from underground, is lined with greenery no matter

what time of year you visit. Blue Spring and the area around it were a lodge and retreat until 1960, when it was purchased by the Missouri Department of Conservation. Rocky Falls and Klepzig Mill are two other must-see sites within easy striking distance of Logyard. Rocky Falls is an example of a shut-in, a place where extremely hard erosion-resistant rock has "shut in" a stream. In this particular shut-in Rocky Creek flows through a layer of rhyolite porphyry, forming a 40-foot cascade with a wonderful swimming hole at its outflow. Picnic sites with tables and grills are here, making Rocky Falls a great place to hang out with your family.

Klepzig Mill, remnants of an early 1900s water-powered turbine mill, is 1.5 miles downstream from Rocky Falls. It was built by Walter Klepzig in 1928 next to another shut-in on Rocky Creek. Two weathered buildings containing old millworks still stand next to the stream, and traces of the old dam and millrace can be spotted in the creek. This haunting spot doesn't have a swimming hole like the one at Rocky Falls, but the cascades

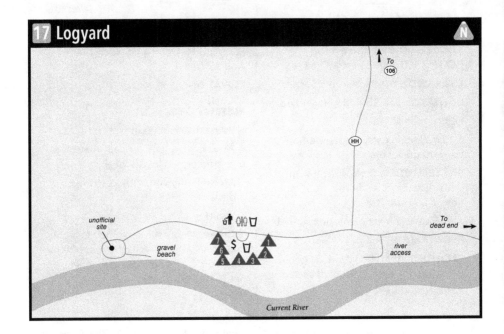

in the shut-in flow through narrow chutes that are perfect for cooling off on a hot summer day in the Ozark Riverways.

Both Rocky Falls and Klepzig Mill can be reached by driving, or on foot via the Ozark Trail. For more information and directions to both sites, read profiles for Powder Mill and Two Rivers (see the next page and page 74, respectively).

:: Getting There

Drive 14 miles west of Ellington on MO 106 to MO HH. Go 6 miles south on MO HH to a T-intersection with a gravel road. Turn right and drive 0.5 mile to Logyard Primitive Camp.

GPS COORDINATES N 37° 6.792' W 91° 7.627'

18

Powder Mill

A 1-mile hike south from Powder Mill leads to spectacular Blue Spring, the deepest of the several Ozark springs sharing that name.

Powder Mill is a small campground on the east bank of the Current River. Shaded by a grove of tall trees that fends off the afternoon sun, this camp is near the old Powder Mill Ferry site. Named for a long-gone mill that once manufactured gunpowder nearby, the ferry was the only local way across the Current until the MO 106 bridge was built in 1975. A rugged bluff towers over the Current north of the MO 106 bridge, and a mile downstream the most beautiful spring in the Ozarks tumbles into the river.

Powder Mill's 10 campsites are scattered along both sides of a tadpole-shaped loop drive. Sites 1–5, lined up along the west side of the camp road, are closest to the Current River. If you're a water bug, these sites are the place to be—they're only a few steps from the stream. All have good afternoon shade except site 5. Sites 6–10, on the road's east side, are better shaded and a little more secluded. Of these, site 6 is my pick. Located at the end of the road, it's the most private spot to pitch your tent at Powder

Mill. Because all sites are close to the Current, this is a fine place to ride out the heat of summer. At Powder Mill the river is wide and calm, which makes it a wonderful place to swim, wade, fish, or sunbathe. Canoeing is still enjoyable near Powder Mill, but because of the deep waters in this stretch of the Current, powerboats will often interrupt your peaceful canoeing reveries.

Powder Mill's best attractions are the nearby hiking trails. The campground is the trailhead for a 1-mile downriver hike to Blue Spring. This level footpath is an easy hike, with views of the sparkling Current River on your right all the way to the spring. You can also reach the spring by driving 2 miles east on MO 106 to a sign directing you to Blue Spring, and then driving another 2.5 miles south on a gravel road.

Regardless of how you get here, you'll be awed by this natural wonder. Although numerous springs in the Ozarks are called Blue Spring, this azure jewel is the bluest of them all. Viewing platforms at the spring's edge and on the low bluff above let you gaze into the pool's 300-foot depths. Each day Blue Spring pours 90 million gallons of water into the Current River.

The Blair Creek section of the Ozark Trail comes down from the north on the Powder Mill side of the river. At MO 106 the trail crosses the bridge, becomes the Current River section, and continues south

:: Ratings

BEAUTY: ★ ★ ★ ★ ★
PRIVACY: ★ ★ ★ ★
SPACIOUSNESS: ★ ★ ★ ★ ★
QUIET: ★ ★ ★ ★ ★
SECURITY: ★ ★ ★ ★
CLEANLINESS: ★ ★ ★ ★ ★

:: Key Information

ADDRESS: 404 Watercress Dr., P.O. Box 490, Van Buren, MO 63965

OPERATED BY: National Park Service

CONTACT: 573-323-4236; nps.gov/ozar

OPEN: Year-round

SITES: 10

SITE AMENITIES: Table, fire pit with grate, lantern pole

ASSIGNMENT: First come, first served

REGISTRATION: Self-pay at campground entrance

FACILITIES: Apr. 16–Oct. 14: Water, flush toilets; Year-round: River access, trails

PARKING: At each site

FEE: Apr. 16–Oct. 14: $12; Oct. 15–Apr. 15: free

ELEVATION: 650'

RESTRICTIONS:

■ **Pets:** On 6-foot leash

■ **Fires:** In fire pits; burn only firewood gathered or purchased locally

■ **Alcohol:** Allowed, subject to local ordinances

■ **Vehicles:** Up to 40 feet

■ **Other:** 14-day stay limit; no glass containers in caves or within 50 feet of river; 6-person, 2-tent limit per site; quiet hours 10 p.m.–6 a.m.

along the river's west side. Both of these sections feature some of the prettiest hiking on the entire Ozark Trail. If you hike a mile north from the bridge, you'll have two wonderful overlooks from bluffs above Owl's Bend of the Current River. You'll see the river streaming by below, the MO 106 bridge, farms on the far side, and the Ozark Mountains marching into the distance.

Though the Current River section showcases wonderful scenery for its entire length, in its northern 10 miles you'll find two must-see sites. Don't miss historic Klepzig Mill, 7 miles from Powder Mill, and Rocky Falls, 9 miles south of Powder Mill. Both are on Rocky Creek, which flows into the Current River 5 miles downstream from Powder Mill.

If you're not up for hiking, you can drive to both sites. To get to Rocky Falls, drive 5 miles west on MO 106 to MO H, turn south, go 5 miles to MO NN, and then head east 2 miles to Rocky Falls. A quarter-mile drive south down a gravel road leads to the falls and a wooded picnic area. Next to the picnic sites, a wide, calm pool stretches downstream

from a steel gray mass of smooth rock over which Rocky Creek tumbles in an incredible display of cascades.

To get to Klepzig Mill, continue east on MO NN until the pavement ends. Take the left fork of two gravel roads and drive about 2 miles to the mill. You're there when you see two unpainted wooden shacks on the right side of the road. These two buildings are what remain from the early 1900s gristmill that once operated on this set of shut-ins and cascades on Rocky Creek. One of the buildings still contains some millworks, and if you work your way around the rocky shut-ins, you'll be able to pick out remains of the long-gone dam and millrace.

If you come to Klepzig Mill when it's hot, you'll enjoy sitting in the smooth rock troughs of the shut-ins and letting the cool water flow over you. To see even more pretty scenery, hike south from the Klepzig Mill on the Ozark Trail. You'll follow Rocky Creek past pools, boulders, low bluffs, and wooded mountains on your way to Rocky Falls. It's a 1.5-mile hike to MO NN and 3 miles to Rocky Falls.

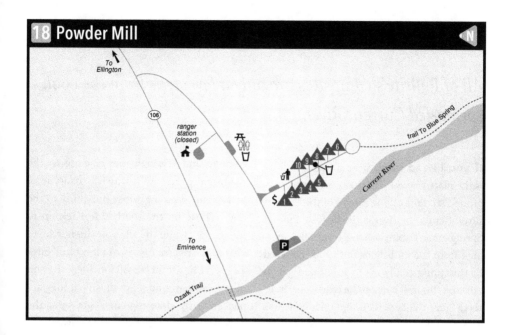

:: Getting There

From Eminence drive 12 miles east on MO 106. The campground entrance is on the right just east of the Current River Bridge.

GPS COORDINATES N 37° 11.441' W 91° 10.321'

19

Pulltite

All of Pulltite's campsites are only a few steps from the cool, spring-fed Current River.

If you like to camp near streams, Pulltite is the place for you. This long, narrow campground stretches along a bend of the Current River. Across the river is the historic Pulltite Spring and Cabin, where gristmills operated from the mid-1800s until 1911. Powered by the spring's daily 20- to 30-million-gallon outflow, this mill deep in the river valley indirectly gave the area its unique name. It was a "tight pull" for mules and horses pulling wagonloads of ground meal from the mill to the hillsides above the village of Pulltite.

Sites are a little crowded and the openness of the area limits privacy, but these disadvantages are offset by the campground's layout. Pulltite's long and narrow configuration keeps it from feeling crowded when it's full. Most sites are level spaces in grassy areas. If you like to be near the action, settle into sites 1–13. They are in a small, well-shaded loop near the river access and campground entrance. A small store and canoe rental service operates next to these sites, and nearby is the campground's new shower house.

Sites 14–42 are located on both sides of the gravel road leading to the back of the

campground. Though they're close to the road, many are excellent, with shade, level grassy tent sites, and close proximity to the river. Those on the south side back up to the woods, while the sites on the north are next to the river across from a low bluff. Sites 44–55 are in another small loop near the end of the campground. Like sites 1–13, they are packed fairly close together. Site 55 at the back of the loop offers the most privacy.

The group sites are the best camping spots at Pulltite. Group Camp 3, at the very end of the campground road, is a remote site right on the river's edge. It is also the trailhead for the 1.5-mile Pulltite Trail, a relatively easy hike following the banks of the Current for a third of its length before climbing into the hills east of the river. On the northeast side of the loop you'll see an intermittent spring trickling from a small box canyon. Just south of the spring is a cave. In summer the cave entrance is a cool place, and on cold winter days it breathes warm moist air on your face.

During your stay at Pulltite be sure to check out Pulltite Spring and Cabin. Because it's across the Current from camp, you'll have to wade or canoe to check out this historic site. Splashing through the cool, spring-fed river is a delight on hot, humid summer days.

Great canoeing awaits you at Pulltite. You can paddle the scenic upper Current River on floats of varying lengths and end up here. Pulltite is 24 miles from Baptist,

:: Ratings

BEAUTY: ★ ★ ★ ★
PRIVACY: ★ ★
SPACIOUSNESS: ★ ★ ★
QUIET: ★ ★ ★
SECURITY: ★ ★ ★ ★
CLEANLINESS: ★ ★ ★ ★ ★

:: Key Information

ADDRESS: 404 Watercress Dr., P.O. Box 490, Van Buren, MO 63965

OPERATED BY: National Park Service

CONTACT: 573-323-4236; nps.gov/ozar

OPEN: Year-round

SITES: 55 individual, 3 group

SITE AMENITIES: Table, fire pit with grate, lantern pole

ASSIGNMENT: First come, first served; reservations required for group sites

REGISTRATION: Self-pay at campground entrance

FACILITIES: Apr. 16–Oct. 14: Water, showers, store; Year-round: Vault toilets, river access, canoe rental, trails

PARKING: At each site

FEE: Apr. 16–Oct. 14: $14 individual, $100 group; Oct. 15–Apr. 15: free

ELEVATION: 740'

RESTRICTIONS:

■ **Pets:** On 6-foot leash

■ **Fires:** In fire pits, rings, or pans; burn only firewood gathered or purchased locally

■ **Alcohol:** Allowed, subject to local ordinances

■ **Vehicles:** No limit, but most sites unsuitable for large RVs

■ **Other:** 14-day stay limit; no glass containers in caves or within 50 feet of river; 6-person, 2-tent limit per site; quiet hours 10 p.m.–6 a.m.

17 miles from Cedargrove, and 10 miles from Akers. If the river's flowing strongly, you could paddle the whole distance from Baptist but wouldn't have time to relax or explore along the way. Current River is best done in sections or as a two-day float.

Take your time on the river, because there are several things you shouldn't miss. One of these is fishing—from Baptist to Akers the cool spring-fed Current contains trout. From Baptist to Cedargrove it's a trophy trout management area, so bring your fly rod and fishing license and start thinking of fishing stories to tell when you get back.

About 5 miles downriver from Baptist you'll see Parker Hollow on your left, where a small creek pours into the Current. A short walk up the hollow leads you to the historic Nichols Cabin, an abandoned Ozarks farmstead restored in the 1980s. It's worth the hike to check out this old farm, and imagine what life must have been like in days past in the Current River Valley.

And 5 river miles below Cedargrove Access is Welch Spring and Hospital, another haunting ruin on the Current. Built over a cave next to a 75-million-gallon-per-day spring, the remains of this early 20th-century hospital are fascinating to explore. An Illinois doctor built the hospital with the belief that spring waters and the cool, clean air from the cave had medicinal healing qualities. Even though his plan didn't pan out, the hospital rooms with views of the Current River flowing past must have made his patients feel a little better.

A half mile downriver from Welch Spring is Welch Landing. Directly across the river from the landing is the Howell-Maggard Cabin Stabilization Project, another abandoned homesite. Restoration of this farmstead began in 2000. Cave Spring is 5 miles below Akers. The pool at the back of the cave is more than 100 feet deep. This spring draws its water from nearby Devils Well, another site you shouldn't miss while camping in the Ozark Riverways.

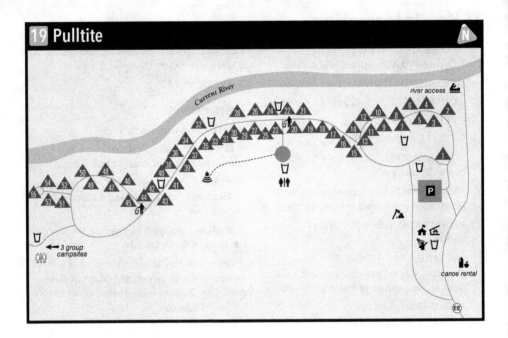

:: Getting There

From Salem drive 25 miles south on MO 19 to MO EE. Turn west on MO EE and follow it 4 miles to Pulltite.

GPS COORDINATES   N 37° 20.074'   W 91° 28.622'

20

Round Spring

Sixty years before it became part of the Ozark National Scenic Riverways, Round Spring was one of Missouri's first state parks.

Long before there was an Ozark National Scenic Riverways, Missourians realized that Round Spring was a treasure. In 1924 this jewel near the banks of the Current River became one of Missouri's first state parks. Named for the shape of the pool from which it flows, Round Spring wells gently from the earth at a rate of 26 million gallons daily, flows through a fissure in the wall surrounding its pool, and meanders into the Current River.

The main campground at Round Spring is beautiful. For a well-developed campground it's a surprisingly laid-back place. Sites are a little close together, but landscaping and thick woods make things feel fairly private. It's built into a hillside above the river, with many sites terraced above or below the camp road, thus creating a more isolated atmosphere. The paved road eliminates dust and the annoying crunch of tires on gravel.

Sites on the main loop road are more private and well shaded. E1–E6, Round Spring's six sites with electricity and water,

:: Ratings

BEAUTY: ★ ★ ★ ★
PRIVACY: ★ ★ ★
SPACIOUSNESS: ★ ★ ★
QUIET: ★ ★ ★ ★
SECURITY: ★ ★ ★ ★
CLEANLINESS: ★ ★ ★ ★ ★

are located on the road that bisects the loop; they are open and poorly shaded. Sites 30–35 are walk-in camping spots. Site 25, with a nice view of the Current River, is my favorite spot at Round Spring.

Across Spring Creek from the main campground are group camps 4–9. They are level and grassy but offer little shade or privacy. Group camps 1–3 are exceptionally nice sites. Away from the other group camps, they're located across the river and the highway, north of the main recreation area, and next to the store and canoe rental service. Situated in shady woods on the river's edge, these three group camps have wonderful sites.

The campgrounds and attractions at Round Spring are connected by a trail paralleling MO 19. This path crosses the Current River and Spring Creek on pedestrian bridges arching high above the streams. The trail is a handy thing—you can hike it from the main campground to the group camps, and then jump into the Current for a half-mile tubing run back to camp.

Although the Ozarks are full of caves, many folks are afraid to venture alone into one. That's not a problem here—just west of the campground is Round Spring Cave, where you can take a tour to admire the underground beauty of the Ozarks. Guided forays into the cave have historically been offered daily June–August, but tours were

:: Key Information

ADDRESS: 404 Watercress Dr., P.O. Box 490, Van Buren, MO 63965

OPERATED BY: National Park Service

CONTACT: 573-323-4236; nps.gov/ozar

OPEN: Year-round

SITES: 54 individual (including 6 walk-in and 6 with water and electric), 9 group

SITE AMENITIES: Table, fire pit with grate, lantern pole

ASSIGNMENT: First come, first served; reservations available at 877-444-6777 or recreation.gov (required for group sites)

REGISTRATION: Self-pay at campground entrance

FACILITIES: Apr. 16–Oct. 14: Water, flush toilets, visitor center, showers, laundry; Year-round: Vault toilets, pavilion, store, river access, canoe rental, trails

PARKING: At each site

FEE: Apr. 16–Oct. 14: $14 individual, $17 with water and electric, $100 group; Oct. 15–Apr. 15: free

ELEVATION: 700'

RESTRICTIONS:

■ **Pets:** On 6-foot leash

■ **Fires:** In fire pits; burn only firewood gathered or purchased locally

■ **Alcohol:** Allowed, subject to local ordinances

■ **Vehicles:** Up to 30 feet

■ **Other:** 14-day stay limit; no glass containers in caves or within 50 feet of river; 6-person, 2-tent limit per site; quiet hours 10 p.m.–6 a.m.

ceased in early 2013 due to the sequester. The National Park Service hopes that this is only temporary—check the Ozark Riverways website for current information about cave tours.

The Current has plenty of bass and sunfish, but for a real angling challenge, head to the upper river. The cold spring waters there support a state-managed trout fishery. Much of the river is inaccessible by road, so you'll have more opportunities if you canoe to your fishing spots. From Baptist Access to Cedargrove the river is a trophy trout management area, where only artificial baits can be used. From Cedargrove to Akers the Current is a regular trout management area. Study and follow all Missouri fishing rules and regulations.

While canoeing the Current, you'll pass Cave Spring about 5 miles downstream from Akers. It draws its water from Devils Well, a must-see while camping in the Ozark Riverways. You can reach the well by driving north from Round Spring on MO 19 to MO KK, and then turning west on KK to a gravel road with a sign directing you 1.5 miles to Devils Well.

Once at Devils Well, you'll see a staircase descending into the bowels of the earth. Sinkholes are all over the Ozarks, but rarely can you enter one. Here you'll go underground and peer into a deep pool 100 feet below. A switch lets you flood the chamber with light to admire the sight of hundreds of water droplets showering from the chamber's ceiling into the pool below.

A must-see historic site near Devils Well is Welch Hospital, built over a cave's mouth next to the 75-million-gallon-per-day flow of Welch Spring. Believing that the moist cave air and clear spring water had medicinal properties, Dr. C. H. Diehl built this hospital in the early 1900s. Two miles north of Akers on MO K and a half mile west on a gravel road is Welch Landing. From there it's a pretty half-mile hike

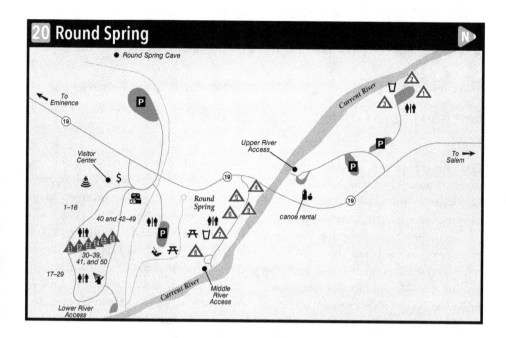

upstream to this abandoned hospital. The spring gurgles from the base of a 25-foot bluff and flows 200 feet to the river. A ledge on the bluff makes a perfect overlook of the hospital ruin and the spring's cascade into the Current River.

Across the river from Welch Landing is the Howell-Maggard Cabin Stabilization Project. The cabin is thought to have been built in the 1850s, and the land around it was farmed by the Howell family until the 1930s. Owned by Earl Maggard until the NPS bought it in 1969, the cabin began undergoing restoration in 2000. Walk around this old homesite and your thoughts will drift back to old times in the Ozarks.

:: Getting There

From Salem drive 30 miles south on MO 19. From Eminence drive 13 miles north on MO 19.

GPS COORDINATES   N 37° 16.843'   W 91° 24.656'

21

Two Rivers

Two Rivers is a laid-back little campground overlooking the junction of the Current and Jacks Fork Rivers.

Two Rivers is the smallest developed campground on the Ozark National Scenic Riverways. With its 22 individual sites and two group camps scattered among the trees, its atmosphere is comfortably intimate. Everything you need for a campout—water, restrooms, showers, river access, and even a small store—is within a few feet of your campsite. The store has a veranda overlooking the junction of the Jacks Fork and Current Rivers, where you can spot fish lolling in a deep hole at the confluence.

While Two Rivers is a compact little place, it doesn't feel crowded even when the camp is full. Mature trees shade the campground, with plenty of open area that gives the place a spacious feel. Most sites on the main loop offer views of the intersection of the rivers, and the spacing is just right—close enough for making friends with your neighbors but far enough to feel comfortably separate.

The 12 campsites on the main loop are all shaded, especially those in the outside of the circle drive. Site 6 is my favorite. It has trees all around it and an open grassy space behind it—ideal for a couple of tents. The only drawback is close proximity to the road, but because there's hardly any traffic and the road is paved, there's little noise and no dust. Site 7 is just like 6, but it's a little too close to the restrooms.

Sites 8, 9, and 10 are at the back of the loop and thus are the most secluded ones on the main loop at Two Rivers. Site 8, with plenty of grassy tent space around it, is the best of these three. Sites 11 and 12, on the right as you enter the loop, are nice sites too. Site 11 is a little rough, but there's a hideaway tent space in the woods behind it. Sites 1–5 are all on the inside of the loop and have plenty of level, grassy tent space all around them. You'll have to be more careful when placing your tent for shade at these sites, but several big trees block these spots from sun much of the day.

Walk-in sites 13–19 are next to the Current River, just downstream from the store. They're in a small open area, tucked against a belt of riverside trees that shade them for much of the day. Sites 18 and 19 are the most secluded of these, but they aren't as level as the other walk-ins. They're spaced just the right distance apart and are so close to their parking area that they're almost like car-camping sites. The walk-ins are great for swimmers—a staircase leads down to the Current River between sites 17 and 18.

My favorite sites here are 20–22, located downstream from the main camp and right

:: Ratings

BEAUTY: ★ ★ ★ ★
PRIVACY: ★ ★ ★
SPACIOUSNESS: ★ ★ ★ ★
QUIET: ★ ★ ★ ★
SECURITY: ★ ★ ★ ★ ★
CLEANLINESS: ★ ★ ★ ★ ★

:: Key Information

ADDRESS: 404 Watercress Dr., P.O. Box 490, Van Buren, MO 63965

OPERATED BY: National Park Service

CONTACT: 573-323-4236; nps.gov/ozar

OPEN: Year-round

SITES: 12 individual, 7 walk-in, 3 back-country, 2 group

SITE AMENITIES: Table (except at back-country sites), fire pit with grate, lantern pole

ASSIGNMENT: First come, first served; reservations required for group sites

REGISTRATION: Self-pay at campground entrance

FACILITIES: Apr. 16–Oct. 14: Water, showers, store; Year-round: Flush toilets, river access, canoe rental

PARKING: At each site

FEE: Apr. 16–Oct. 14: $14 individual, $100 group, $5 for 3 riverside sites; Oct. 15–Apr. 15: free

ELEVATION: 660'

RESTRICTIONS:
- **Pets:** On 6-foot leash
- **Fires:** In fire pits; burn only firewood gathered or purchased locally
- **Alcohol:** Allowed, subject to local ordinances
- **Vehicles:** Up to 20 feet
- **Other:** 14-day stay limit; no glass containers in caves or within 50 feet of river; 6-person, 2-tent limit per site; quiet hours 10 p.m.–6 a.m.

on the river's edge. Because their access road crosses deep gravel deposits left by the river when it runs high, getting to these sites can be a bit dicey without four-wheel drive. I made it in my little Mazda 626, though, so whatever you're driving, just put your foot on the gas and go for it. It's worth the adventure—these are among the most scenic and secluded official campsites in the entire Ozark Riverways. Because they're considered backcountry campsites, their fee is only $5, payable at the signboard just west of the river access. Each site has a lantern pole, fire pit, grill, and trash can, but no table. Watch the weather—a rising river would quickly overrun these streamside campsites.

Two Rivers is a nice place to end a canoe trip. You come off the river only a few steps from your campsite and walk past a store stocked with snacks and cold drinks—a nice treat after a day on the water. If you haven't had enough of the river for one day, you can go back there to fish for smallmouth bass.

Several other attractions are within a short drive of Two Rivers, and all of them can be combined with hikes. One of these is Blue Spring, just downstream from Powder Mill Campground where MO 106 crosses the Current. Possibly the prettiest spring in the Ozarks, Blue Spring can be reached via a 1-mile riverside hike from Powder Mill, or by driving 2 miles beyond it, and then heading 2.5 miles south on a marked gravel road. Ninety million gallons flow daily from its azure depths and rush over beds of watercress to the Current River a few feet away. Platforms above the spring offer views far into its mysterious depths.

Another nearby spot is Rocky Falls, an incredible display of cascades in Rocky Creek. You can drive right to Rocky Falls, and picnic sites with views of the falls await you there. A calm pool below the falls reflects the rocky, tree-covered hillside, and you can climb to the top of the cascade and dangle your feet in tumbling waters. To get there

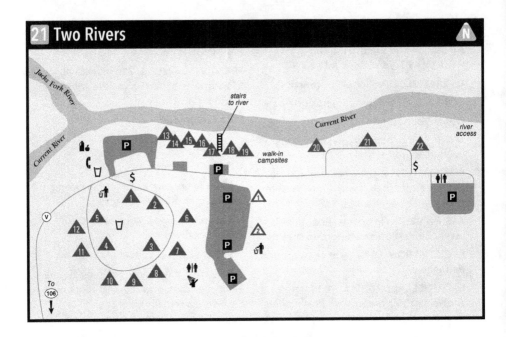

from Two Rivers, go back out to MO 106, drive 2.5 miles east to MO H, go 5 miles south on MO H to MO NN, and then turn east 2 miles on MO NN to the gravel entrance drive to Rocky Falls.

The Ozark Trail passes near Rocky Falls, and a spur trail leads from the falls to the trail. A 3-mile hike north on the Ozark Trail is Klepzig Mill, the abandoned remnants of an early 1900s gristmill on Rocky Creek. You'll find the sunbaked remains of

a couple of buildings, some old millworks, and the foundations of the mill's dam and raceway. The creek flows over a set of shut-ins next to the mill, and on a hot day it's fun to sit in one of the cool, frothy troughs or cascades in this haunting old mill site. Nonhikers can drive to the mill. From Rocky Falls, continue east on MO NN until the pavement ends at a forked gravel road. Take the left fork, and 2 miles later you'll reach the old mill.

:: Getting There

From Eminence drive 5 miles east on MO 106 to MO V. Turn left on MO V and follow it 3 miles to Two Rivers.

GPS COORDINATES   N 37° 11.380'   W 91° 16.599'

Mark Twain National Forest

22

Berryman Recreation Area

This pine-shaded hideaway is the trailhead for the Berryman Trail, the most popular backcountry mountain biking ride in Missouri.

Berryman Recreation Area is the old campsite of Civilian Conservation Corps Company 3733. The picnic pavilion here is dedicated to the men who worked at the camp in the 1930s. Berryman Campground is a wonderful place to hang out. A mixture of mature pines and hardwoods shades all the sites, and on rainy days you can walk over to the picnic shelter to continue reading, writing, relaxing, or shooting the breeze with fellow campers. There's a nice open lawn near the shelter for sun worshippers, who enjoy soaking up some sun even on those cool and crisp fall days that are such a delight in the Ozarks. The lawn is a superb place for stargazing too, making Berryman a great camp for observing special astronomical events such as comets, lunar eclipses, or one of the several meteor showers that light up the heavens each year.

Berryman is a good place for active folks too—the Ozark Trail goes through the camp, running all the way to Taum Sauk

Mountain State Park and the Eleven Point River in the south, and north to Onondaga Cave State Park. The Ozark Trail is still under construction, and the Ozark Trail Association hopes to one day connect it to the Ozark Highlands Trail in northwest Arkansas. The Berryman Trail, a 24-mile loop popular with hikers, mountain bikers, and equestrians, also passes through the campground. It's the most popular mountain biking route in Missouri and has been written up in numerous national publications. And for those hot days when it's too muggy to bike or hike, you can canoe on nearby Huzzah and Courtois Creeks, two of Missouri's nicest float streams.

Berryman's eight sites aren't numbered in any way. They're laid out like a tadpole, with four sites forming the tadpole's head and four scattered along its tail. All sites are spaced well apart from each other, and because all are excellent camping spots shaded by thick forest, it's hard to pick a favorite. The ones on the turnaround loop are farthest from the middle of this recreation area, but the camp is such a quiet place that those searching for solitude will find it at any site at Berryman. The only criteria I can think of for choosing a site at Berryman is proximity to the restrooms. They're at the beginning of the campground, just before the first site, and the farther back you camp, the longer your late-night excursions will be. This little hideaway rarely fills,

:: Ratings

BEAUTY: ★ ★ ★ ★
PRIVACY: ★ ★ ★ ★
SPACIOUSNESS: ★ ★ ★ ★
QUIET: ★ ★ ★ ★ ★
SECURITY: ★ ★ ★ ★
CLEANLINESS: ★ ★ ★ ★

:: Key Information

ADDRESS: 10019 W. MO 8,
P.O. Box 188, Potosi, MO 63664

OPERATED BY: Mark Twain NF/Potosi/
Fredericktown Ranger District

CONTACT: 573-438-5427;
www.fs.usda.gov/mtnf

OPEN: Year-round

SITES: 8

SITE AMENITIES: Table, lantern pole,
fire pit with grate

ASSIGNMENT: First come, first served

REGISTRATION: None required

FACILITIES: Vault toilets, pavilion, picnic
sites, trails; no water available

PARKING: At each site

FEE: Free

ELEVATION: 1,000'

RESTRICTIONS:

■ **Pets:** On leash only

■ **Fires:** In fire pits; burn only wood
gathered or purchased locally

■ **Alcohol:** Allowed, subject to local
ordinances

■ **Vehicles:** Up to 25 feet

■ **Other:** 14-day stay limit

so it's always a peaceful place—and with no fee, it's one of the real camping deals in the Ozarks. The camp's only drawback is its lack of drinking water, so bring plenty.

Berryman's big attraction is the Berryman Trail. It's a longtime favorite with hikers, but since the advent of the mountain bike, this trail has become the most popular backcountry mountain bike adventure in Missouri. Some short trails near the urban areas get more use, but the Berryman is known around the region as the trail to pedal in the Show Me State. With many climbs, rock-strewn technical sections, and a satisfying length, the Berryman is ideal for experienced riders. It's a tough ride for novices, but beginners with a good attitude will like the Berryman very much. Because numerous road crossings make good places to bail out, the trail is good for beginners to try their first backcountry singletrack challenge.

Almost all of the Berryman Trail is singletrack. Some stretches are rough and rocky, but few will require portaging your bike. Because the trail alternates between ridgetops and creek bottoms, the scenery includes both pleasant meandering streams and views from the tops of the climbs. The trail is partially carved out of the shoulders of ridges, skirting deep, quiet hollows in the forest, often meandering through groves of tall pines that sway and sigh in ridgetop breezes.

Your ride will swoop around the tops of hollows, plunge to valley floors, and pass two springs. One of these, Edward Beecher Spring, is a fascinating trail highlight. Actually an artesian well, Beecher is in a pretty meadow. An iron casing with a pipe extending from the side of the well constantly disgorges cool, clear water into a small trough. It's a nice place for lunch on your excursion. The spring looks clear and clean, but you should purify its water if you intend to drink it. Beecher is about 6 miles north from Berryman Campground and 2 miles south of the Forest Service Road 2265 crossing.

The Berryman also makes a great hike. You can do it in one day, but only if you work like a dog. Most hikers doing the entire trail make it a two- or three-day backpack trip. My favorite day hike uses the northern part of the trail, starting from Brazil Creek Trailhead near the end of MO W, 6 miles north

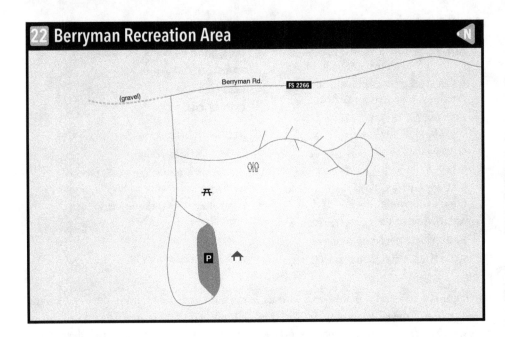

22 Berryman Recreation Area

Berryman Rd.

FS 2266

(gravel)

of Berryman Campground. Hike 1.5 miles up MO W from Brazil Creek to where the pavement ends at FS 2265. About 100 feet past there, pick up the trail where it crosses FS 2265, turn right, and hike back to camp. On the way you'll pass by Harmon Spring, wander through quiet hillside pine groves, and end the 8-mile loop hike by descending steeply back to Brazil Creek on a nice set of switchbacks.

:: Getting There

From Potosi drive 17 miles west on MO 8 to Forest Service Road 2266/Berryman Road/County Road 207. Turn north and drive 1 mile to the campground on the left side of the road.

GPS COORDINATES   N 37° 55.775'   W 91° 3.718'

23

Council Bluff
Recreation Area

The trail around Council Bluff Lake connects to the Ozark Trail, opening up miles of backcountry hiking and biking.

Council Bluff Recreation Area is built around 440-acre Council Bluff Lake on the Big River. Opened in 1985, Wild Boar Ridge Campground is a group of campsites strung along the spine of a forested Ozark ridge above the lake. Stretching over a mile-long ridge instead of being crammed into the tight cluster we've come to expect in public campgrounds, sites in Wild Boar Campground are comfortably spaced. All have ample level space for tents. Though many sites are large enough for RVs, the lack of hookups keeps most RVs away. When a behemoth does show up, good spacing between sites and thick woods between camps keep things private and peaceful.

The most secluded sites are the nine walk-ins. They have all the amenities of the vehicle sites but are tucked back in the woods off the main loop and spaced at least 100 feet apart. The most secluded vehicle sites are 25–35 at the far end of the road. My favorite is site 32 at the very end.

:: Ratings

BEAUTY: ★ ★ ★ ★
PRIVACY: ★ ★ ★ ★ ★
SPACIOUSNESS: ★ ★ ★ ★
QUIET: ★ ★ ★ ★ ★
SECURITY: ★ ★ ★ ★ ★
CLEANLINESS: ★ ★ ★ ★ ★

No matter where you camp, you're never far from the water faucets and restrooms scattered throughout this well-designed campground. I especially like the cooking shelters at all sites. They're little but have shelves big enough to store your cooking gear, covered with just enough roof to protect you and your grub from downpours while you whip up your outdoor cuisine. When it's clear, you won't need any shelter from the hot sun—all sites are heavily shaded.

I think even being lazy at Council Bluff is fun. Take a book out to the beach and relax on the sand. Drag your lawn chair to one of the small promontories on the lake's edge and listen to the waves lapping at the shore. Watch the trees around the campsite sway in the ridgetop breezes.

Feeling a little more active? Take a swim at Chapel Hill Beach and Picnic Area. The sandy beach is perfect for bare feet, and the lake is clear and sparkling blue. You can walk the 3 miles from Wild Boar Campground to the beach on the Council Bluff Trail. Those wanting a longer excursion can hike all the way around the lake on this 12.5-mile path. In many places it follows the shoreline, with constant views of blue water and green hillsides. Snags stretching up out of the water in the coves serve as roosts for woodpeckers, kingfishers, herons, and the occasional hawk or osprey. The trail doesn't

:: Key Information

ADDRESS: 10019 MO 8 W., P.O. Box 188, Potosi, MO 63664

OPERATED BY: Mark Twain NF/Potosi/Fredericktown Ranger District

CONTACT: 573-438-5427; www.fs.usda.gov/mtnf

OPEN: Year-round

SITES: 39 individual, 7 double, 9 walk-in, 4 group

SITE AMENITIES: Picnic table, fire pit with grate, lantern pole, cooking shelter

ASSIGNMENT: First come, first served; reservations at 877-444-6777 or recreation.gov

REGISTRATION: Pay host at site 2

FACILITIES: Water, vault toilets, picnic area, pavilion, horseshoe pits, trails, boat ramp, beach (Memorial Day–Labor Day)

PARKING: At site; separate lots for walk-in sites; $3 day-use fee per vehicle at boat ramp, trailhead, and beach

FEE: $10 individual, $20 double, $25 group; $9 nonrefundable reservation fee

ELEVATION: 1,300'

RESTRICTIONS:

■ **Pets:** On leash only; no pets on beach

■ **Fires:** In fire pits; burn only wood gathered or purchased locally

■ **Alcohol:** Allowed, subject to local ordinances

■ **Vehicles:** Up to 40 feet

■ **Other:** 14-day stay limit; no glass containers or coolers on beach

have a lot of ups and downs, so it's not too difficult to hike.

The Council Bluff Trail is open to mountain bikes too. It has become a favorite ride for cyclists out of St. Louis. While it is a moderate trail for hiking, it's a tough bike ride. Though there isn't a lot of climbing, the rocky and rugged surface requires good bike-handling skills and will shake you up a little. If you're a novice, just ride the part between the campground and the beach—it's not too hard and is the prettiest stretch. Two spur trails connect the campground to the trail. One spur leaves the camp road next to the horseshoe pits, and the other drops off the ridge at the end of the campground road.

The Ozark Trail passes within a half mile of Council Bluff Lake. A half-mile spur along Telleck Branch connects it to the Council Bluff Trail, opening up miles and miles of Ozarks hiking and biking. For another good novice ride, follow the Council Bluff Trail from the campground to the connector trail, and then follow it west to the Ozark Trail. Turn north on the Ozark Trail and follow it north to MO DD, where you can turn right and ride the highway and Council Bluff Recreation Area roads back to the campground to complete a 6-mile loop.

If you tire of the trails in Council Bluff, check out the nearby Bell Mountain Wilderness Area, where a 5-mile one-way hike will take you to Missouri's second-highest point. Use the Ottery Creek Trailhead for the Ozark Trail on MO A, 6 miles south of MO 32. From Ottery Creek, the first mile of the Ozark Trail switchbacks steeply uphill, opening up vistas that make the trip worthwhile. Just over a mile up the mountainside the trail forks, and the Ozark Trail bears right. Take the left fork and continue uphill, climbing gradually to the top of Bell Mountain, 1,702 feet above sea level. It's a

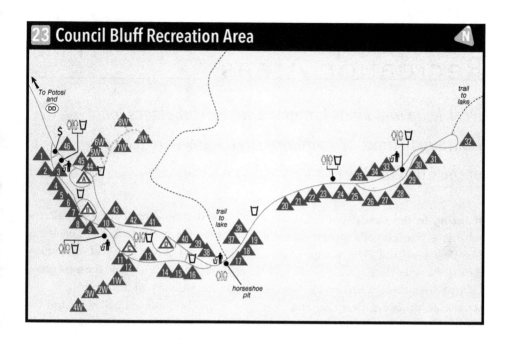

tough climb, but along the way you'll enjoy long-distance vistas from open glades on an impressive boulder-strewn plateau. Once off the Ozark Trail, the route isn't marked, so it's a good idea to bring a map or Missouri hiking guide.

:: Getting There

From Potosi drive 13 miles south on MO P to MO C. Go west on MO C a quarter mile to MO DD. On MO DD go south 7 miles to Council Bluff Recreation Area and follow the signs 1.8 miles to Wild Boar Ridge Campground.

GPS COORDINATES   N 37° 43.881'   W 90° 56.765'

24

Deer Leap and Float Camp Recreation Areas

Deer Leap and Float Camp are wonderful places for floating, fishing, or swimming in the lower reaches of the Current River.

If lazing in the shade next to a beautiful river is your idea of a good time, you'll like Deer Leap and Float Camp. Located next to the wide, deep reaches of the lower Current River, these camps are comfortable streamside hideaways. Deer Leap and Float Camp are two separate recreation areas in the Mark Twain National Forest. Because they're only a half mile apart, I decided to lump them together as a single campground. Both camps were renovated in 2011–2012, making them a little more developed than I'd normally prefer, but they're still wonderful places to pitch your tent.

Float Camp is the best loop for families. Its 20 sites are in an open area shaded with tall hardwoods. A small playground entertains kids, while older folks gravitate to the horseshoe pits. When Float Camp was renovated its loop road and parking spurs were widened and paved, and gravel pads were laid for the tents and picnic tables. Sites 1–4 and 16–20 at the beginning of the loop are electric and are more suitable for RVs. Nonelectric sites 5–17 are on the back half of the loop, and of these, sites 10–15 have the most grassy space for pitching your tent.

This flat-bottomed hollow next to the Current River is a wonderful enclave, with room to toss a Frisbee or play catch. The river is only a few steps away, and a gently sloping gravel beach makes this a great wading and swimming hole. A shady path crosses a bridge between the campground and the beach, passing through a small alcove in the woods with benches overlooking the river. The alcove is a wonderful spot to admire the river and watch the kids as they splash in the stream.

A nice riverside path leads from camp to the picnic area. There you'll find a shelter, picnic sites, more swimming, changing rooms, and a sand volleyball court. The water is deeper near the picnic area, with hidden drop-offs, so be careful.

Deer Leap, with only 10 sites, is quieter and more private than Float Camp. Its sites are a little farther apart and are separated by belts of woods. Deer Leap doesn't have nice swimming areas like Float Camp, and it lacks amenities such as picnic sites, pavilions, and volleyball courts. Consequently, while both of these cool and shady riverside

:: Ratings

BEAUTY: ★ ★ ★ ★
PRIVACY: ★ ★ ★
SPACIOUSNESS: ★ ★ ★ ★ ★
QUIET: ★ ★ ★ ★
SECURITY: ★ ★ ★ ★
CLEANLINESS: ★ ★ ★ ★ ★

:: Key Information

ADDRESS: #4 Confederate Ridge Rd., Doniphan, MO 63935

OPERATED BY: Mark Twain NF/Eleven Point Ranger District; KC's on the Current

CONTACT: 573-996-2153; www.fs.usda .gov/mtnf; kcsonthecurrent.com

OPEN: Apr.-Sept.

SITES: 30

SITE AMENITIES: Table, fire pit with grate, lantern pole; some in Float Camp have cooking shelters and electricity

ASSIGNMENT: First come, first served

REGISTRATION: Self-pay at loop entrances

FACILITIES: Water, vault toilets, river access; Float Camp: Picnic area, pavilion, playground, volleyball nets, horseshoe pits, trails

PARKING: At each site; $3 per vehicle in day-use areas

FEE: $12 single, $18 double, $20 single electric, $30 double electric

ELEVATION: 350'

RESTRICTIONS:

■ **Pets:** On leash only

■ **Fires:** In fire pits; burn only wood gathered or purchased locally

■ **Alcohol:** Allowed, subject to local ordinances

■ **Vehicles:** Up to 34 feet at Deer Leap; up to 60 feet at Float Camp

■ **Other:** 14-day stay limit; 8-person limit per site; quiet hours 10 p.m.-6 a.m.; no glass containers at swimming areas; no fireworks

camps may be full on hot summer weekends, Deer Leap is likely to be the more peaceful of the two. Site 10, at the end of the campground road right at the river's edge, is my favorite site at Deer Leap.

The blue waters of the Current make these camping loops wonderful summer hangouts. Tubing is a great way to enjoy the campgrounds. At Float Camp, use the trail between the picnic area and campground for short runs without a shuttle. You can do the same at Deer Leap, bobbing along the river from the head of the campground to the river access for a half-mile run, and walking the road back to camp. Using a shuttle driver lets you float the Current from site 9 at Deer Leap to the camping loop at Float Camp on a 1-mile tubing run. Wear life jackets—here in its lower reaches the river's current is strong.

While this part of the Current River is tamer than its upper reaches in the Ozark National Scenic Riverways, it still offers great canoeing. Fewer gravel bars and obstructions make it a better float for families with small children. It's an easy 5-mile paddle to Doniphan, where you can have an ice cream cone before heading back to camp. Local outfitters can shuttle you upriver for longer trips back to your campsite at Float Camp and Deer Leap. The wider and deeper reaches of the lower Current offer excellent fishing, so bring along your fishing gear and go after the bass, sunfish, buffalo fish, and catfish that hide in the river below your canoe.

Two short trails at Float Camp explore the forest around the campground. The half-mile Woodchuck Trail follows the river between the camp and the day-use area and then climbs the hills above to overlook the Current. The 1.5-mile White Oak Trail explores the hills east of the campground. Near the trailhead at the picnic area, the

24 Deer Leap and Float Camp Recreation Areas

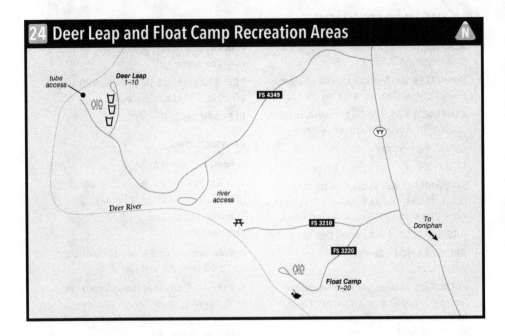

White Oak Trail passes Malden Spring. Though not as impressive as its brothers Alley, Greer, and Big Springs, Malden is still a pretty little trickle pouring 8,000 gallons daily into the Current River.

KC's on the Current, located in nearby Doniphan, manages both campgrounds for the U. S. Forest Service and can outfit you for floating, tubing, or fishing while you're enjoying the Ozarks at Deer Leap and Float Camp Recreation Areas. Check them out at **kcsonthecurrent.com.**

:: Getting There

Take MO YY 4.5 miles north of Doniphan. Deer Leap's entrance is a half mile past Float Camp. Both are on the west side of the highway.

GPS COORDINATES   **Deer Leap** N 36° 40.690'   W 90° 52.017'
                      Float Camp N 36° 40.179'   W 90° 51.914'

25

Dry Fork Recreation Area

Dry Fork is a quiet, laid-back campground on the 35-mile Cedar Creek Trail.

Dry Fork Recreation Area is a peaceful campground on the northern edge of the Missouri Ozarks. The landscape around Dry Fork is a transition zone where forest gives way to grassland, featuring a mix of oak, hickory, and pine trees with scattered prairie openings. Consequently, you'll see a variety of wildlife in this diverse terrain. From your campsite at Dry Fork you can explore this interesting landscape on the 35-mile Cedar Creek Trail System. A network of three loops open to hikers, mountain bikers, and equestrians, the Cedar Creek Trail runs past the camp. Dry Fork is also only a short drive from the Katy Trail, a scenic 225-mile rails-to-trails conversion running from Clinton to St. Charles.

Dry Fork Camp lacks the stately pines and grassy spaces that adorn its sister camp a few miles away at Pine Ridge, but it's attractive in its own way. Its eight private sites are tucked into groves of cedars in the surrounding oak-hickory-pine forest, and a pine-shaded picnic area is just up the road from camp. Hidden away on a gravel road in the

forest, the camp is a nice quiet place to spend a few days. All its sites are well spaced, private, and shady. Best of all, the campground is open year-round on a donation-only basis, and unlike many other campgrounds in Missouri, frost-free hydrants let the water stay on all year long.

If you're an equestrian, you'll really like Dry Fork. All sites have hitching posts, and a spur leads from camp to the Cedar Creek Trail, a popular central Missouri riding destination. If you're not into horses, Dry Fork is still a fine place to be—when I camped there, I was impressed with how well the riders had cleaned up after their horses. They were really good neighbors too—not a single road apple could be found at Dry Fork after they left. Signs on the hitching posts ask equestrians to remove their straw and pony pucks to a disposal area across the road, and they do an excellent job of complying.

Sites 1–4 on the east side of the loop are the best sites at Dry Fork. The cedar groves are at their thickest around these spacious level sites. Site 1 is my favorite camping spot—an old cemetery separates this nook in the cedars from the other spots on this side of the loop, and water is right next to the site. I don't get lonely there—when night falls, ghosts from the cemetery come keep me company. Sites 2, 3, and 4 are well spaced, and gaps in the cedars allowing access from one to the other make these good sites for families or small groups.

:: Ratings

BEAUTY: ★ ★ ★
PRIVACY: ★ ★ ★ ★ ★
SPACIOUSNESS: ★ ★ ★ ★
QUIET: ★ ★ ★ ★ ★
SECURITY: ★ ★ ★ ★
CLEANLINESS: ★ ★ ★ ★

:: Key Information

ADDRESS: 4549 MO H, Fulton, MO 65251

OPERATED BY: Mark Twain NF/Houston/Rolla/Cedar Creek Ranger District

CONTACT: 573-592-1400; www.fs.usda.gov/mtnf

OPEN: Year-round

SITES: 8

SITE AMENITIES: Table, lantern pole, fire grate, hitching post

ASSIGNMENT: First come, first served

REGISTRATION: Self-registration at entrance

FACILITIES: Water, vault toilets, picnic sites, trail

PARKING: At each site

FEE: Donations accepted

ELEVATION: 780'

RESTRICTIONS:

■ **Pets:** On leash only

■ **Fires:** In fire pits; burn only wood gathered or purchased locally

■ **Alcohol:** Allowed, subject to local ordinances

■ **Vehicles:** Up to 34 feet

■ **Other:** 14-day stay limit

Beyond site 4 is the vault toilet, and behind it is the spur path to the Cedar Creek Trail. Sites 5, 6, and 7 are all nice camping spots, but not quite as pretty as sites 1–4. Site 8, an average site at best, is the only unattractive camping spot at Dry Fork.

The Cedar Creek Trail, a popular ride for both equestrians and mountain bikers that passes by Dry Fork, is divided into three sections. The 22-mile main loop is the original Cedar Creek Trail, and it's the part that goes by the camp. The 7-mile Moon Loop, the northernmost part of the network, is named for the eroded landscape through which it passes. The 5-mile Smith Creek Loop explores a 1,500-acre semiprimitive area between Cedar Creek and MO J. The Cedar Creek Trail is too long a ride for many bikers, but carrying a forest map of the Cedar Creek District lets you use numerous road crossings to choose loops of varying lengths for riders of differing skill and endurance levels. Where the north side of the main loop crosses Cedar Creek, you'll find Rutherford Bridge, an abandoned steel span across which a local scout troop has constructed a footbridge.

Though the Cedar Creek Trail is a bit long for day hiking, a good short trek is the 4 miles between Dry Fork and Pine Ridge Recreation Areas. A 3-mile hike south from Dry Fork leads to the Nevins Homestead, two stabilized buildings from an old farmstead that's being slowly reclaimed by the forest. The area around the farm looks so hardscrabble that it's hard to imagine wresting a living from this challenging landscape, but the Nevins family was able to make a go of it here.

If you're into fishing, visit Carrington Pits Recreation Area northeast of Dry Fork. Carrington Pits is 3 miles west of Fulton on MO H, and then 1 mile north on County Road 315. It's a beautiful set of ponds formed in abandoned strip pits from a long-ago coal mining operation. Now filled with water and surrounded by cedars and hardwoods, these ponds are stocked with largemouth bass, sunfish, and catfish. There are picnic sites for hanging out, and a trail leads to two fishing piers on the old, now-scenic strip pond.

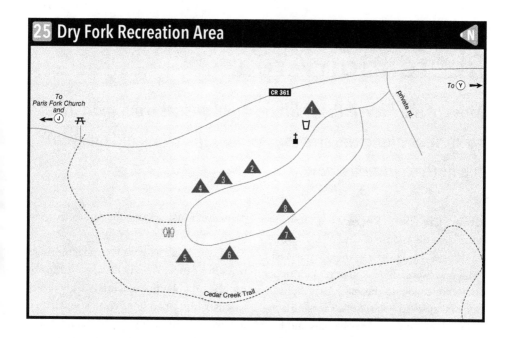

:: Getting There

From Ashland drive 8 miles east on MO Y to County Road 363. Turn north and follow this gravel road 1.5 miles to CR 361. Turn right and follow CR 361 0.7 mile to
the camp entrance on the left side of the road. From I-70 Exit 137, go south 12 miles
on MO J to CR 356, where there's a sign for the Paris Fork Methodist Church. Go
right (west) 1.2 miles to CR 361, and then drive south 1.2 miles to the camp.

GPS COORDINATES   N 38° 47.003'   W 92° 7.523'

26

Greer Crossing Recreation Area

Most of the Eleven Point River's flow gushes from more than 30 springs along the stream, keeping the river cold on even the hottest summer day.

Greer Crossing Recreation Area is smack in the middle of one of my favorite landscapes in Missouri—the Eleven Point Wild and Scenic River country. With upper access for canoeing the most beautiful section of the Eleven Point, Greer Crossing is the perfect base for exploring the hills and hollows near the river. Located a few hundred feet from the river, Greer's sites are level, well spaced, and shady. Most of these spacious grassy sites have room for two or more tents. Walls of trees and brush separate you from the neighbors. No sites are directly on the Eleven Point, but it's only a short walk to a dip at the nearby picnic area and river access.

The water is refreshing, but you'll be out in a hurry—most of the Eleven Point's flow gushes from the 30 springs that feed it, keeping the river cold on the hottest summer day. Put on your waders and come back, though, because the cool water provides a rare pleasure in the Midwest—a wild-trout population just waiting for you to try your hand at fly-fishing.

If you don't have waders, go after those trout in a canoe. Whether you are fishing or just drifting along, canoeing is a good way to enjoy this sparkling, clear stream. Just upstream from camp, Greer Spring pours 220 million gallons daily into the Eleven Point, so you'll have good river levels no matter how dry the season. The best stretch to float begins at Greer Crossing and runs 19 miles to Riverton. It's most enjoyable as a two-day trip with an overnight at one of the six float camps along the river.

All the float camps are nice, but White's Creek, located in the 16,500-acre Irish Wilderness, is my favorite. From the camp you can explore this remote wildland on the White's Creek Trail. A half-mile hike along the south side of the loop goes to the mouth of White's Creek Cave, a cool 1,600-foot-long cavern with many impressive formations. The cave is closed for now to protect bat populations, but you can still lean against its gate on a hot day and relax in its cooling breath. Hiking 3 miles north from White's Creek Camp, you'll meander through the woods to a quarter-mile section of trail on a bluff above the river, where there's a spectacular overlook of Bliss Spring flowing into the Eleven Point.

:: Ratings

BEAUTY: ★ ★ ★ ★ ★
PRIVACY: ★ ★ ★ ★
SPACIOUSNESS: ★ ★ ★ ★ ★
QUIET: ★ ★ ★ ★
SECURITY: ★ ★ ★ ★
CLEANLINESS: ★ ★ ★ ★ ★

:: Key Information

ADDRESS: Route 1, Box 1908 MO 19 N., Winona, MO 65588

OPERATED BY: Mark Twain NF/Eleven Point Ranger District

CONTACT: 573-325-4233; www.fs.usda.gov/mtnf

OPEN: Year-round

SITES: 20

SITE AMENITIES: Table, fire pit with grate, lantern pole; sites 9 and 13 have cooking shelters

ASSIGNMENT: First come, first served

REGISTRATION: Self-registration at loop entrance

FACILITIES: May–mid-Oct.: Water;

Year-round: Vault toilets, picnic areas, river access, trails

PARKING: At each site

FEE: $10 single, $15 double

ELEVATION: 530'

RESTRICTIONS:

■ **Pets:** On leash only

■ **Fires:** In fire grates; burn only wood gathered or purchased locally

■ **Alcohol:** Allowed, subject to local ordinances

■ **Vehicles:** Up to 60 feet

■ **Other:** 14-day stay limit; no glass containers within 50 feet of river

If canoeing isn't your thing, there are other great trails around camp that you don't need a boat to access. You can hike the Irish Wilderness from Camp Five Pond Trailhead on MO J. It's about 7 miles from the pond to White's Creek. You can hike or mountain bike right from your campsite on the Ozark Trail. The Ozark Trail runs over 100 miles northeast from Greer Crossing, passing through the Ozark National Scenic Riverways and extending all the way to Onondaga Cave State Park. If it's a short hike you want, take the easy 1-mile trail to exquisite Greer Spring. Its trailhead is on MO 19, 1.5 miles south of the campground.

Turner Mill Access is a haunting and historic spot on the Eleven Point. Accessible by either canoe or car, Turner Mill was once the location of Surprise, a village named for the residents' reaction to approval of a post office application for their remote village. The community was born in the 1850s when G. W. Decker tapped a spring that flowed from a cave to power his mill next to the Eleven Point. In 1891 Jesse L. Clay Turner

bought the mill, refurbished it into a four-story structure, and operated it well into the 1900s. Turner also ran a general store, built a bridge over the river, provided land and materials for the Surprise School, and hired its teacher.

Little is left of Surprise today, but interpretive signs at the site tell the settlement's story and display a photo of the mill in its heyday. The spring still gurgles from a cave in the low bluff overlooking the mill site, and the 25-foot steel, overshot mill wheel, quiet for the last 60 years, stands like a ghost in the spring branch. The Surprise School still stands in the woods 100 yards downriver—its blackboard and outhouses still in place. Its last graduating class matriculated in 1945. The path to the school starts near the upper end of Turner Mill's parking area.

Turner Mill Access is 5 miles downriver by canoe or 11 miles by car on a combination of paved and gravel roads. Turner Mill makes a nice mountain bike ride too. Pedal the Ozark Trail 10 miles east from

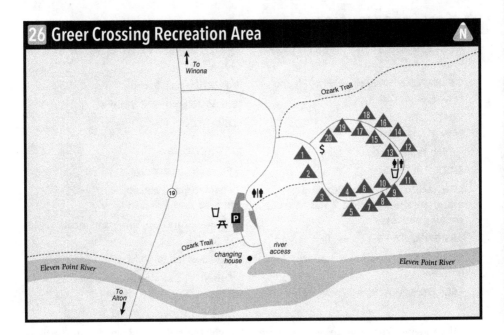

Greer Crossing to the trailhead on Forest Service Road 3152. Take FS 3152 a half mile east to FS 3190, and go south on FS 3190 to Turner Mill. A snack and a splash in the river at Turner Mill are the perfect boost for a return to Greer Crossing via roads for a 24-mile loop.

For more outdoor adventures in the Eleven Point area, check out McCormack Lake Recreation Area on page 105.

:: Getting There

From Winona take MO 19 south for 17 miles. The recreation area entrance is on the east side of the road just before the bridge over the Eleven Point River.

GPS COORDINATES   N 36° 47.691'   W 91° 19.799'

27

Lane Spring Recreation Area

Beautiful Lane Spring, with its parklike setting, is a popular place for weddings.

Lane Spring Recreation Area is a pleasant little spot for an afternoon or weekend escape. Though it's close to the city of Rolla, it's a hidden enclave in the valley of Little Piney Creek that feels like the middle of nowhere. Completely renovated in 1996, the picnic area and campground are wonderful places to relax and enjoy the outdoors. Lane Spring is great for families or other groups too—the picnic area has pavilions for reunions, a playground for kids, and a field big enough for softball games or tossing a Frisbee around.

The campground is well separated from the picnic area, ensuring a peaceful camping experience no matter how many day users are in the park area. Sites 1–5 and site 7 have electricity. Most sites are separated from their neighbors by 100 feet or so, with thick walls of trees and brush bolstering their privacy. Many of the 18 campsites border Little Piney Creek, with paths leading out to the creek's gravel bars and cooling water. The gurgling of the stream will lull you to sleep by night and invite you to drag your lawn chair and cold drink to its shores

:: Ratings

BEAUTY: ★ ★ ★ ★
PRIVACY: ★ ★ ★ ★
SPACIOUSNESS: ★ ★ ★ ★
QUIET: ★ ★ ★ ★ ★
SECURITY: ★ ★ ★ ★
CLEANLINESS: ★ ★ ★ ★ ★

by day. Tall pines and hardwoods shade all of the sites.

Little Piney Creek, fed by numerous springs, is a clear and chilly little stream. Four of these springs—Lane, Yancy Mills, Twin, and Table Rock—flow into the creek near camp. Lane Spring, located in the picnic area, is a magical place. Stonework walls, walks, and steps surround this little bubbler and the branch that flows from the spring over to Little Piney Creek. In fact, many couples from Rolla and other surrounding towns come here for weddings and portraits.

From the stone overlook above Lane Spring, you can see the spring bubbling into the bottom of the pool. Fine silt dancing in the boils looks like delicate brown flowers or tiny volcanoes on the bottom of the pool and spring branch. Brilliant green watercress grows in the crystal-clear spring water, adding vivid color to the scene even in winter.

Follow the stone steps to the water's edge, where the spring branch pours into Little Piney Creek. The spring-fed creek is a wonderful place to wade or swim on hot and humid summer days. Gravel bars, instream boulders, and cool, clear water make the creek a wonderful place to explore or just hang out enjoying nature's beauty.

Fly-fishing is an excellent way to enjoy Little Piney Creek. Above and below Lane Spring Recreation Area, trout thrive in the cool water from the numerous springs feeding the Little Piney. In many places the creek

:: Key Information

ADDRESS: 401 Fairgrounds Rd., Rolla, MO 65401

OPERATED BY: Mark Twain NF/Houston/Rolla/Cedar Creek Ranger District

CONTACT: 573-364-4621; www.fs.usda.gov/mtnf

OPEN: Apr.–Oct.; gate may be closed 10 p.m.–6 a.m.

SITES: 17 individual, 1 double

SITE AMENITIES: Table, lantern pole, fire pit with grate

ASSIGNMENT: First come, first served

REGISTRATION: Self-pay at loop entrance

FACILITIES: Water, vault toilets, pavilions, picnic sites, playground, trails

PARKING: At each site

FEE: $8 individual, $16 double, $15 electric, $34 pavilion; $2 day-use fee per vehicle

ELEVATION: 820'

RESTRICTIONS:

■ **Pets:** On leash only; not allowed in the creek

■ **Fires:** In fire pits; burn only wood gathered or purchased locally

■ **Alcohol:** Allowed, subject to local ordinances

■ **Vehicles**: Up to 34 feet

■ **Other:** 14-day stay limit; no glass containers in Little Piney Creek

is wide enough for back casting, which makes it a good place for novice fly-fishermen.

Even if you don't hook anything, working your way up and down Little Piney Creek and letting your rod and reel pull you deeper into the outdoors is a fun way to spend an afternoon. I've often wondered who's getting caught—the fish by the fisherman, or the angler by the outdoors. Probably a little of both, just as it should be.

Hiking is another way to be pulled deeper into the outdoors at Lane Spring. Two trails built by Boy Scouts from Rolla explore the land above and along Little Piney Creek. The easier Cedar Bluff Trail covers 1.5 miles. It begins next to the picnic area and climbs to a rocky glade near a bluff overlooking the valley of the creek. Bring your binoculars and enjoy the view, and then follow the trail as it descends back to creek level and follows the bottomlands back to Lane Spring.

The 1-mile Blossom Rock Trail is a tougher hike but well worth your effort. You can start this hike behind the pay station

or from a spur trail in the campground near sites 16 and 17. You'll climb high onto a bluff above Little Piney Creek and pass a huge sandstone boulder that gives the trail its name. This monster of a rock, 50 feet tall and 125 feet across, has cracks and lines that make its surface seem to blossom. From Blossom Rock the trail descends steeply to the bottoms, where you'll follow the creek back to the campground.

Other activities nearby include mountain biking and canoeing. Little Piney Creek flows into the Gasconade River not far from where its cousin, the Big Piney River, also joins the Gasconade. Both the Big Piney and the Gasconade are fine canoeing streams, with put-ins within 20–30 miles from Lane Spring. Just south of Newburg is the Kaintuck Trail, a network offering hiking and biking loops of 1–15 miles. Its trailhead is in Mill Creek Picnic Area, where another trout fishery thrives. You won't run out of things to do in this part of the Mark Twain National Forest.

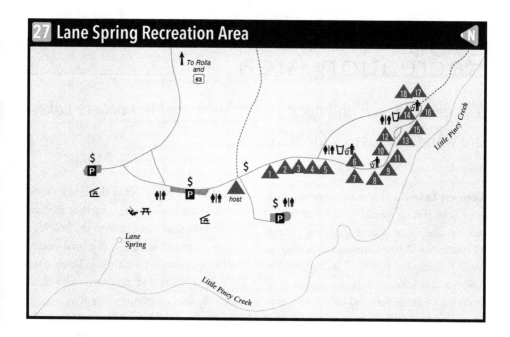

:: Getting There

From Rolla drive 11 miles south on US 63 to Forest Service Road 1892, where you'll see a sign for Lane Spring Recreation Area. Turn west and drive 1.4 miles to the recreation area. Turn left by the picnic area at the bottom of the hill and follow the signs a short distance to the campground.

GPS COORDINATES N 37° 47.946' W 91° 48.938'

28

Loggers Lake Recreation Area

The gravel beach and open grassy lawn next to Loggers Lake are wonderful places for stargazing.

Loggers Lake is one of many beautiful facilities built throughout Missouri and Arkansas by the Great Depression–era Civilian Conservation Corps. Constructed in 1939–40 by CCC Company 1730 from nearby Bunker, Loggers Lake is a clear blue, 22-acre pool surrounded by green-forested hills. The campground at this end-of-the-road hideaway is a peaceful Ozarks retreat and a great place to hike, swim, boat, fish, or simply relax.

Coming down the big hill to Loggers Lake, you first arrive at a pretty picnic area on a small peninsula to your right. Next you splash through Mill Creek on a slab bridge, curve around the lake, pass another picnic area and the beach, and enter the campground. Sites 1–4 are above the beach and below the road. They're a bit close to the pavement, but being set 6 feet below road level makes them feel more secluded. Sites 5 and 6, down a short spur road right next to the lake, are very nice camping spots. They have the best view of the lake and are

:: Ratings

BEAUTY: ★ ★ ★ ★
PRIVACY: ★ ★ ★
SPACIOUSNESS: ★ ★ ★ ★
QUIET: ★ ★ ★ ★ ★
SECURITY: ★ ★ ★ ★
CLEANLINESS: ★ ★ ★ ★ ★

shaded by tall pines. All of the first six sites are packed a little tightly together but are wonderfully shady and close to the beach.

Just beyond sites 1–6 the road enters the loop containing sites 7–14. These sites are farther apart and more spacious than sites 1–6. All except sites 9 and 14 are on the outside of the loop with good distances between them. The loop is in a grassy open area with fewer trees than sites 1–6, giving each site a nice view of the lake. Sites 10–13 are closest to the water. Because the road is paved, all sites are free of dust and that annoying rattle of tires on gravel. With plenty of space for a couple of tents, these sites are better for small groups.

This wonderful, laid-back campground is great for hanging out. Next to the picnic area is a small gravel beach ideal for swimming and wading. Loggers Lake is a nice place to drift around in your canoe too. Whether from a canoe or the lake's shores, anglers can go after smallmouth bass and sunfish. The beach and the more open campsites in the loop make great places for soaking up some sun or doing a little late-night stargazing.

If you feel more active, you can hike two trails from the camp at Loggers Lake. A short 0.3-mile trail leads from the slab bridge over Mill Creek to Rock Springs, a small bubbler that helps Mill Creek keep

:: Key Information

ADDRESS: 1301 S. Main St., Salem, MO 65560

OPERATED BY: Mark Twain NF/Salem Ranger District

CONTACT: 573-729-6656; www.fs.usda.gov/mtnf

OPEN: Apr.–Oct.; walk-in only Nov.–Mar.

SITES: 14

SITE AMENITIES: Table, fire pit with grate; most with lantern pole

ASSIGNMENT: First come, first served

REGISTRATION: Self-pay at loop entrance

FACILITIES: Apr.–Oct.: Water, picnic area, swimming beach, boat ramp, horseshoe pits, trail; Year-round: Vault toilets

PARKING: At each site; $2 day-use fee per vehicle for noncampers

FEE: $8

ELEVATION: 1,020'

RESTRICTIONS:

■ **Pets:** On leash only

■ **Fires:** In fire pits; burn only wood gathered or purchased locally

■ **Alcohol:** Allowed, subject to local ordinances

■ **Vehicles:** Up to 34 feet

■ **Other:** 14-day stay limit; no glass containers on swimming beach; quiet hours 10 p.m.–6 a.m.

the lake filled with cool water. A longer hike is the 1.5-mile Loggers Lake Nature Trail, a pretty tramp around the lakeshore. The trail starts behind site 13, where you'll find a trailhead and wooden sign with an etched route map. This loop hike crosses the dam, passes through tall oaks and pines, and has a spur to the now-closed Oak Knoll Campground located on a ridge above the lake.

You can do some longer hiking and a bit of mountain biking on the nearby Ozark Trail, just 10 miles to the east. A trailhead is located 3 miles southeast of Bunker, at the junction of MO 72 and MO P. This trailhead is the southwestern end of the 25-mile Karkaghne section of the Ozark Trail and the northern terminus of the 27-mile Blair Creek section. The Karkaghne is open to mountain bikers and hikers, and its southwestern end offers the easiest bicycling on this section. You can make a nice 7-mile loop by riding from the trailhead east to MO TT, passing through a huge grove of old-growth evergreens in Vest Hollow, and then returning to the trailhead via MO TT and MO 72.

The Blair Creek section parallels MO P, intersecting it 3 miles south of the trailhead. It follows a ridgetop between Blair and Big Creeks with few difficult ups and downs. You can do a nice 6-mile loop by hiking the trail until it crosses MO P and then walking the little-traveled highway back to the trailhead. If you hike the entire Blair Creek section of the Ozark Trail, you'll enjoy spectacular views at its southern end.

A short drive west takes you to the upper reaches of the Current River in the Ozark National Scenic Riverways. Loggers Lake is a nice base for exploration of the Ozark Riverways, as its campsites are inexpensive and uncrowded. At Akers Ferry, 25 miles west of Loggers Lake at the junction of MO K and MO KK, you can ride an old ferry across the upper Current River. You can also rent a canoe and check out this river from the seat

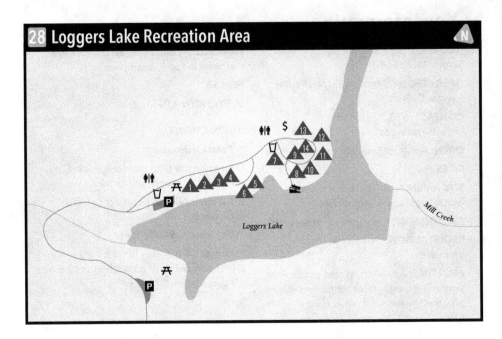

28 Loggers Lake Recreation Area

Loggers Lake

Mill Creek

of your boat. Not far south of Akers are the fascinating sites of Devil's Well, a sinkhole that feeds the Current River, and Welch Hospital, the ruins of an abandoned health spa built upon the mouth of Welch Spring. Pick up an Ozark Riverways map at Akers and explore these haunting places along the Current River.

:: Getting There

From the intersection of MO 72/MO A in Bunker, drive 0.5 mile west on MO A to Lincoln Avenue (sign points southwest to Loggers Lake). Lincoln Avenue changes to gravel and becomes County Road 565. Follow CR 565 for 6 miles to Forest Service Road 2193. Turn south and go 1 mile to Loggers Lake.

GPS COORDINATES   N 37° 23.735'   W 91° 16.430'

29

Marble Creek Recreation Area

The pond behind the old mill dam on Marble Creek
is sparkling, clear, and inviting.

Marble Creek is named for the pinkish dolomite called Taum Sauk marble. This marble is found along the creek's 20-mile course through the surrounding St. Francois Mountains. Like so many Ozark streams, the creek was once harnessed to power a mill. In Marble Creek Recreation Area you can swim in the old mill pool and examine crumbling foundations of a mill that last operated in the 1930s. This laid-back streamside campground is a quiet hideaway for tent camping.

The campground is nestled in a horseshoe bend of Marble Creek with a pleasant blend of thick woods and open tree cover. Sites on the back half of the loop are farther apart and are separated by thick bands of brush, while those near the front of the campground are more open and parklike. The best sites are 11, 13, and 15. Located on the back of the loop, they're on ledges overlooking the stream. Site 17 is a good one too—it's at creek level and is a great place for wading and splashing in Marble Creek.

In the front half of the campground

:: Ratings

BEAUTY: ★ ★ ★ ★
PRIVACY: ★ ★ ★ ★
SPACIOUSNESS: ★ ★ ★ ★ ★
QUIET: ★ ★ ★ ★
SECURITY: ★ ★ ★ ★
CLEANLINESS: ★ ★ ★ ★ ★

several sites on the east side of the loop are set back in the trees with a grassy meadow behind them. They're good spots for larger groups or families. So are the sites on the inside of the campground's loop road, where scattered hardwoods and pines shade spacious grassy spots. With its mix of open sites and shaded streamside camping spots, Marble Creek has a campsite to please everyone.

The picnic area and the millpond are west of the campground loop. The pool is deep, clear, and inviting. Rocks for sunbathing are everywhere up and down this rugged little creek. Bring your rod and reel—smallmouth and rock bass can be caught in the millpond and other pools along Marble Creek. The creek is especially pretty in spring, when heavier flows make this little stream rush and ripple, lulling you to sleep each evening.

Just east of the campground is Lower Rock Creek, one of Missouri's most beautiful wild places. Also known as Dark Hollow or Cathedral Canyon, it's a rugged defile in the St. Francois Mountains, where Lower Rock Creek crashes over boulders and ledges on its way to the St. Francois River. In several spots bluffs tower 400 feet above the rocky streambed. An easy mile-long walk on an old washed-out road leads from the trailhead to the canyon, where you'll find an exquisite place to hang out among pools and cascades. More beauty awaits upstream,

:: Key Information

ADDRESS: 10019 W. MO 8, P.O. Box 188, Potosi, MO 63664

OPERATED BY: Mark Twain NF/Potosi/Fredericktown Ranger District

CONTACT: 573-438-5427; www.fs.usda.gov/mtnf

OPEN: Apr. 15–Oct. 30

SITES: 26

SITE AMENITIES: Table, fire pit with grate, lantern pole

ASSIGNMENT: First come, first served

REGISTRATION: Self-pay at loop entrance

FACILITIES: Apr.–Oct.: Trash; Year-round: Vault toilets, swimming hole, trails; no water available

PARKING: At each site; $2 day-use fee per vehicle for noncampers

FEE: $10 individual, $20 double

ELEVATION: 660'

RESTRICTIONS:

■ **Pets:** On leash only

■ **Fires:** In fire pits; burn only wood gathered or purchased locally

■ **Alcohol:** Allowed, subject to local ordinances

■ **Vehicles:** Up to 25 feet

■ **Other:** 14-day stay limit; no glass containers near swimming hole or creek

but it's a rugged hike among rocks and boulders—and well worth the effort. To reach Lower Rock Creek's trailhead go 7 miles east on MO E to County Road 511, and then go left 0.4 mile and cross a concrete slab bridge. Turn left just past the bridge on a primitive road and follow it 0.4 mile to a locked gate. The abandoned road on the other side leads to Lower Rock Creek.

For a longer trek, head west from camp on the Ozark Trail. The Marble Creek section of the OT starts from a trailhead at the campground entrance, crosses MO E, and runs 8 miles southwest to Crane Lake. Open to both hikers and mountain bikers, this trail is a good introduction to the St. Francois Mountains. It alternately climbs to scenic ridgetops and descends into cool, wooded hollows. Halfway to Crane Lake the trail meanders through a set of rugged, rocky glades with fine vistas of the surrounding mountains.

Upon reaching Crane Lake, the Ozark Trail connects to the 5-mile Crane Lake Trail built by the U.S. Forest Service and the Youth Conservation Corps in the 1970s. The trail around the lake is divided into a 3-mile northern loop and a 2-mile southern loop, with the dam as the cutoff route. This trek follows the lake's edge in some places and climbs to blue-water vistas in others. Below the dam, Crane Pond Creek rushes through a series of shut-ins, pools, and waterfalls in Reader Hollow. Near the junction of the two trails, a spring gurgles from the rocks and joins Crane Pond Creek.

If you bike to Crane Lake, it's easy to turn the ride into a loop by returning to Marble Creek via gravel roads and MO E. Ride 2 miles north on the gravel road leading away from Crane Lake, and turn right at the intersection there. Follow that road 2.5 miles to MO E, and then turn right on MO E and proceed 4 miles to Marble Creek. If you're driving from Marble Creek to Crane to shuttle hikers or pick up cyclists, just reverse the directions. A sign on MO E directs you to Crane Lake.

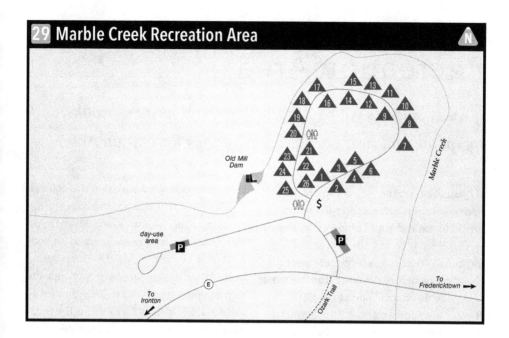

29 Marble Creek Recreation Area

Crane is a national forest picnic site, with tables scattered in the woods next to the lake. It's fun to go to Crane and hike the trail and enjoy a picnic. Bring your fishing pole—the lake is stocked with bass, sunfish, and catfish. Maybe you can catch your supper there.

:: Getting There

Drive 2 miles south of Fredericktown on US 67 to MO E. Turn west on MO E and drive 18 miles to Marble Creek Recreation Area. It will be on the right, immediately after the bridge crossing Marble Creek.

GPS COORDINATES   N 37° 26.969'   W 90° 32.398'

30

Markham Springs Recreation Area

If water soothes your soul, you'll love the springs, brooks, millpond, and river at Markham Springs Recreation Area.

If you like water, you'll love Markham Springs. A deep, clear, spring-fed pool with an old home and a mill house on its shores is the centerpiece of the recreation area. Little brooks trickle everywhere near the pond and picnic area, flowing from the pool and a couple of small springs in this valley. If you want your streams a little bigger, the Black River flows along the back side of the campground loops. Two-and-a-half miles of scenic trails, complete with numerous footbridges across the spring streams, are great for showing you around this pretty hideaway next to the Black River.

A few years ago the Black River badly flooded Markham Springs. The floodwaters damaged the campsites quite a bit, but the U.S. Forest Service and campground hosts have been working hard to restore the place. When I visited in spring 2012, restoration was continuing, but I thought it was already a wonderful place to camp. Several sites were being removed or rearranged, so don't be surprised if there are a few inaccuracies in the campground description that follows.

The best tent sites at Markham Springs are in the Pine, Sycamore, and River Loops. Pine Loop, containing sites 1–12, is on your right as you drive along the campground road. All of its sites are very nice, but the pick camping spot is site 6. It's right next to the Black River. Sites 13–25 are in the Sycamore Loop, the next set of campsites along the park road. Sycamore is a mirror image of Pine Loop, with shady, level, well-spaced sites separated by thin curtains of brush. Site 18, closest to the Black River with a view of the stream, is the best site in Sycamore Loop. Sites 26–40 in the River Loop, located farthest from the camp center, are the most remote sites at Markham Springs.

Birch Loop contains electric sites 41–52. Six of this loop's sites are doubles, and most are shaded. If you like a little open space, Birch Loop is the place. Its sites are arranged around a small grassy meadow, with ample room to toss a Frisbee or spread a blanket to read and relax in the sun. The campground's bathroom and shower house are located on Birch Loop's south end.

Markham Springs Recreation Area is a wonderful woodland hangout. The picturesque valley's scenery is best enjoyed on a leisurely walk from your campsite. The stone home next to the millpond was built in the 1930s and received electricity from a mill wheel powered by the pool's outflow.

:: Ratings

BEAUTY: ★ ★ ★ ★ ★
PRIVACY: ★ ★ ★ ★
SPACIOUSNESS: ★ ★ ★ ★
QUIET: ★ ★ ★ ★
SECURITY: ★ ★ ★ ★
CLEANLINESS: ★ ★ ★ ★ ★

:: Key Information

ADDRESS: 1420 Maud St., Poplar Bluff, MO 63901

OPERATED BY: Mark Twain NF/Poplar Bluff Ranger District

CONTACT: 573-785-1475; markhamsprings.com

OPEN: May 1–Oct. 1

SITES: 40 basic, 12 electric

SITE AMENITIES: Table, fire pit with grate, lantern pole

ASSIGNMENT: First come, first served

REGISTRATION: Self-pay at entrance

FACILITIES: Water, showers, vault toilets, dump station, picnic area, river access, horseshoe pits, volleyball net, trails

PARKING: At each site; $2 day-use fee per vehicle for noncampers

FEE: $10 single, $15 single electric, $18 double, $30 double electric

ELEVATION: 400'

RESTRICTIONS:

- **Pets:** On leash only
- **Fires:** In fire pits; burn only wood gathered or purchased locally
- **Alcohol:** Allowed, subject to local ordinances
- **Vehicles:** Up to 34 feet
- **Other:** 14-day stay limit; no swimming in spring pools and streams; no glass containers in river

If camping is not your thing, you can stay in this five-room stone home. Named the Fuchs House after its builder, it was restored in 2010. Rental rates, along with a fascinating history of Markham Springs, are at **markhamsprings.com.**

The millhouse and waterwheel still stand at the south end of the pond. Paths and bridges spanning the brooks make for delightful exploration of the area south of the spring pool. Near the pond you'll find Bubble Spring, a small trickle gurgling from the earth and feeding a small stream. Little boils of sand in the bottom of a clear pool mark the spring's outflow. South of the spring and millpond is Island Picnic Area, a shaded narrow tract of land between two spring branches. Island is a wonderful place to read, write, or nap on a blanket in the grass.

It's a nice hike on the Eagle Bluff Trail onto the ridge above camp, where you'll enjoy views of the Black River Valley. The trail starts near the boat launch and climbs high above Markham Spring on rough steps,

and then follows the ridge north. Halfway along the ridgeline you can shorten your hike by taking a cutoff trail leading down to the millpond. If you continue north, you'll eventually descend to river level and follow the stream back to the campground in Sycamore Loop. There you can pick up the River Trail and follow it all the way downstream to the boat launch.

If you're feeling really energetic, load up your mountain bike before heading to Markham Springs. Three nearby trails, all within easy drives of the campground, offer 65 miles of knobby-tired fun. Just a few miles to the south is the 22-mile Victory section of the Ozark Trail. It's a point-to-point ride that can be made into a loop by combining sections of trail with gravel forest roads.

The southern trailhead for the Lake Wappapello section of the Ozark Trail is 12 miles away on MO 172 just east of US 67. Of its 31-mile length, the southernmost 15 miles offer the easiest riding. This trail has a connector to the Lake Wappapello Trail in Lake Wappapello State Park, a 15-mile loop ride

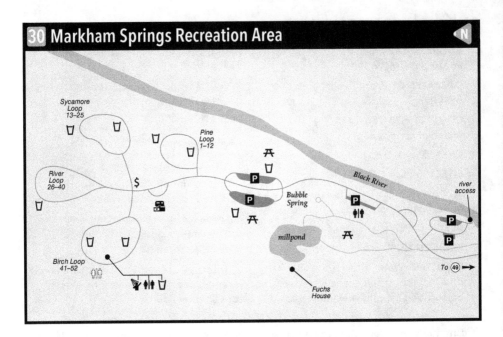

30 Markham Springs Recreation Area

along the lakeshore and through the hills and hollows to the lake's west.

There's one weekend each year when every site at Markham Springs fills, and that's for the Old Tyme Country Festival, held the Saturday after Memorial Day. You might not be able to get a campsite, but come down anyway for live music, crafts, food, antique car and tractor shows, games for the kids, and more. Bring your own guitar, banjo, or fiddle—jams will be going during the festival and on into the night.

:: Getting There

From Williamsville drive 3 miles west on MO 49. The entrance will be on the north side of the road, just after you cross the Black River. The campground is at the back of the recreation area.

GPS COORDINATES N 36° 58.340' W 90° 35.855'

31

McCormack Lake Recreation Area

While you're camping out in Eleven Point River country, don't miss hiking to the incomparable Greer Spring.

Set next to a 15-acre lake built by the Civilian Conservation Corps, McCormack Lake Recreation Area is a quiet and relaxing hideaway. While McCormack isn't spectacular like many of the campgrounds in the Ozarks, it's a peaceful, comfortable place at the end of the road. Because McCormack has only eight sites, it doesn't get crowded and noisy, yet it's only a short distance from the Eleven Point River and its great canoeing and fishing. McCormack Lake itself offers good angling, and great hiking and mountain biking trails leave right from your campsite. McCormack Lake is a little rustic—its toilet, for example, is an open-air fenced enclosure—but it's a free camp, one of the last good deals in the outdoors.

Only six of McCormack's eight sites are regularly used. Sites 1 and 2 are not level, so their tables are usually appropriated and moved to more suitable sites. The other six sites are spacious. Sites 4 and 5 next to the water are the prime spots here. All sites are grassy and shaded by large hardwoods. In

:: Ratings

BEAUTY: ★ ★ ★ ★
PRIVACY: ★ ★ ★
SPACIOUSNESS: ★ ★ ★ ★
QUIET: ★ ★ ★ ★ ★
SECURITY: ★ ★ ★ ★
CLEANLINESS: ★ ★ ★ ★

this small, open campground under the trees, you can see all your neighbors, but adequate distances between sites keep the place from seeming crowded. Summer here can be a little buggy, but in spring the lake's frogs serenade you to sleep, and in fall the lake's waters reflect the autumn colors decorating the surrounding hills.

McCormack Lake is great for both hikers and bikers. If you just want a warm-up or quick sunrise or sunset walk, there is a quarter-mile trail around the lake. For the more energetic, walk the 3.7-mile McCormack-Greer Trail. From the dam it follows McCormack Hollow down to the Eleven Point River and joins the Ozark Trail. It then climbs onto a bluff nearly 300 feet above the river to the Boomhole View, which provides grand vistas up and down this National Wild and Scenic River. During turn-of-the-20th-century logging days, a wooden chute on the bluff across the river was used to slide huge logs down to the Eleven Point, where they landed in the stream with a loud, booming splash.

From the Boomhole the trail descends into Duncan Hollow and forks. Both forks go to Greer Crossing, but the left option climbs onto a ridge and follows it above the Eleven Point, while the easier right path hugs the riverbank. On the river trail you'll see Greer Spring Branch pouring into the Eleven Point, more than doubling the river's size. It

:: Key Information

ADDRESS: Route 1, Box 1908 MO 19 N., Winona, MO 65588

OPERATED BY: Mark Twain NF/Eleven Point Ranger District

CONTACT: 573-325-4233; www.fs.usda.gov/mtnf

OPEN: Year-round

SITES: 8

SITE AMENITIES: Table, lantern pole, fire pit with grate

ASSIGNMENT: First come, first served

REGISTRATION: None required

FACILITIES: Vault toilets, picnic area, trails; no water available

PARKING: At each site

FEE: Free

ELEVATION: 600'

RESTRICTIONS:

■ **Pets:** On leash only

■ **Fires:** In fire pits; burn only wood gathered or purchased locally

■ **Alcohol:** Allowed, subject to local ordinances

■ **Vehicles:** Up to 20 feet

■ **Other:** 14-day stay limit

---

also provides cold water needed to support a trout population, so bring your fly rod.

Greer Spring, from which the branch flows, is a must-see. A 1-mile trail leads to this natural wonder. To take this hike, drive 1.5 miles south of Greer Crossing on MO 19 to a trailhead on the west side of the road. Greer is the second-largest spring in Missouri, gushing 220 million gallons daily into the Eleven Point. From a stone overlook you'll admire the deep blue-green boil of the main spring to your right and a smaller flow emanating from Greer Spring Cave to your left. No matter how hot the day, it's always cool down next to the spring and its 55° outflow.

The natural beauty of Greer Spring and the surrounding forest make it hard to picture this spot as a beehive of activity in the late 1800s. Samuel Greer first built a mill at the spring in 1860. As the forest was logged and farms sprung up in the area, the mill used Greer Spring's power to saw lumber, grind corn, and gin cotton. In 1883 Greer built a new dam and rebuilt the mill

on the hilltop north of the spring, using a cable system to transmit power from the wheel at the spring to the mill above.

The mill finally shut down in 1920, and two years later the Dennig family bought the spring and the land around it. The Dennigs took incredibly good care of the spring for almost 70 years, and then sold it in the late 1980s. The Mark Twain National Forest acquired this natural gem in 1993 through an Anheuser-Busch grant to the River Network and money donated by conservationist Leo Drey. The Dennig family has control of the 110 acres near the spring, where the old mill still stands. Please do not trespass on their land while checking out the spring.

Another attraction near McCormack Lake is Falling Spring Picnic Area. To get there, drive 3 miles north of McCormack Lake on MO 19 to Forest Service Road 3164. Go east on FS 3164, taking the left fork just off the highway, and drive 2 miles to the picnic area. Falling Spring pours 500,000 gallons per day from a rock wall to a pool 20

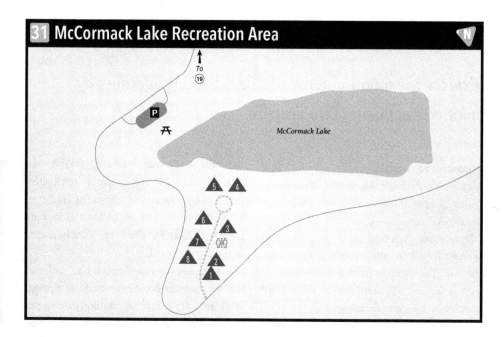

feet below. Beneath the spring you'll see the ruins of another old mill. A short path and footbridge lead to the fascinating piece of history. See the Greer Crossing profile on page 90 for still more trails and attractions in the Eleven Point River country.

:: Getting There

From Winona drive 13 miles south on MO 19 to FS 3155. Turn right on Forest Service Road 3155 and drive 2 miles to the recreation area.

GPS COORDINATES   N 36° 49.322'   W 91° 21.184'

32

North Fork Recreation Area

Explore the 6,600-acre Devil's Backbone Wilderness by hiking or canoeing into deep hills and hollows.

Known to locals as Hammond Mill Camp, North Fork Recreation Area overlooks another of Missouri's many cool, clear, spring-fed streams—the North Fork of the White River. A spring pours into the river a short hike from the far end of the campground. The picnic area and river access are at the far end of camp, where a low bluff overlooks an exceptional spot for a swim during the dog days of an Ozarks summer. The 6,600-acre Devil's Backbone Wilderness wraps around camp to the east, south, and west, and the Ridge Runner Trail heads north from the trailhead near the picnic area. Whether you hike, mountain bike, canoe, or just hang out, you can be as busy or as lazy as you want in this Ozarks haven.

The campground is laid out in three loops hanging like tadpoles off the main road. The sites on the tails of the tadpoles are most private, while those on the turnaround that forms each tadpole's head are a little closer together. The first of these is Dogwood Loop (sites 1–6), with the campground host in site 1. Sites 7–14 are in Willow Loop. With the most sites of the three loops, Willow is a little crowded, but trees separate most sites. Pine Loop is the farthest from the entrance, with sites 15–20. Site 20, at the end of Pine Loop with a view of the river, is the best spot in the campground.

Just past the Pine Loop is the trailhead for the quarter-mile hike to Blue Spring. With an average flow of 7 million gallons per day, it's not huge like Greer or Alley Springs, but this exquisite blue-green pool a few feet from the North Fork is still an Ozarks gem. My friend Janet, who grew up in nearby West Plains, used to bring unsuspecting friends to the campground to go tubing. She'd lure them to the riverside next to the spring, just to hear them gasp and squeal as they drifted unknowingly into the cold outflow.

The spring trail follows the river's edge on the way out to Blue Spring and climbs gently onto hillsides above the stream on the return to the trailhead. It meanders past fascinating rock outcrops, along ledges, and over old stone steps and bridges, with benches along the way for relaxing at the scenic spots. At the spring it skirts the pool's edge, where you can admire the gently roiling surface, and then climbs on top of a small bluff above the spring so you can peer into the blue-green depths. My favorite view is from the short trail running downriver 100 feet from the overlook, where there's a nice vista of the North Fork winding into the forested hills of the Devil's Backbone Wilderness.

:: Ratings

BEAUTY: ★ ★ ★ ★ ★
PRIVACY: ★ ★ ★ ★
SPACIOUSNESS: ★ ★ ★ ★
QUIET: ★ ★ ★ ★
SECURITY: ★ ★ ★ ★
CLEANLINESS: ★ ★ ★ ★ ★

:: Key Information

ADDRESS: 1103 S. Jefferson, Ava, MO 65608

OPERATED BY: Mark Twain NF/Ava/Cassville/Willow Springs Ranger District

CONTACT: 417-683-4428; www.fs.usda.gov/mtnf

OPEN: May 15–Dec. 1

SITES: 20

SITE AMENITIES: Table, fire pit with grate, lantern pole, cooking shelter

ASSIGNMENT: First come, first served

REGISTRATION: Self-pay at entrance

FACILITIES: Water, vault toilets, picnic area, trails, river access

PARKING: At each site; $2 per vehicle day-use fee

FEE: $10 per site; site 1 (electric) $15 when not occupied by host

ELEVATION: 700'

RESTRICTIONS:

■ **Pets:** On leash only

■ **Fires:** In fire pits; burn only wood gathered or purchased locally

■ **Alcohol:** Allowed, subject to local ordinances

■ **Vehicles:** Up to 30 feet

■ **Other:** 14-day stay limit; quiet hours 10 p.m.–6 a.m.

You can explore Devil's Backbone from the Blue Spring Trail. Looping back to camp uphill behind the spring, a trail breaks off to the south. Follow this path a quarter mile uphill onto McGarr Ridge, and you'll intersect one of the trails that wander through this lovely wilderness area. Turn right, and the trail descends over the next mile to a scenic bend in the North Fork. From there, you can swing south and east to follow the trail up Crooked Creek, with optional side trips to McGarr Spring to the north and the Devil's Backbone, a steep-sided narrow ridge, to the south. The trail eventually meanders around the north part of the wilderness, passes a spur leading to a trailhead on MO CC east of the campground, and returns to the Blue Spring spur for a very pretty 9-mile loop.

The Ridge Runner Trail, open to both hikers and mountain bikers, leaves the campground to the north from the trailhead between the camp and the picnic area. On the map it looks like a barbell, with a southern loop near the campground and a long connector going north to another loop at Noblett Lake Recreation Area. The Noblett Loop is 8 miles long and is more rugged than the southern loop. It's a great hike but a difficult mountain bike ride.

The 12-mile North Fork Loop, north of the campground, offers a pleasant hike through wooded hills and is a good intermediate mountain bike ride. I like the west side of the trail best. It hugs the river in a quarter-mile stretch and climbs up high above the North Fork for some nice views of the North Fork valley. When you're next to the North Fork, keep an eye out for river otters—they were recently reintroduced here and are doing well.

When you tire of hiking, rent a tube or canoe and float the North Fork of the White River. Twin Bridges to the North Fork Campground is an easy 5-mile float. If you paddle 4 miles past camp to North Fork Spring, bring your fly rod—you'll be in trout waters for the next 12 miles.

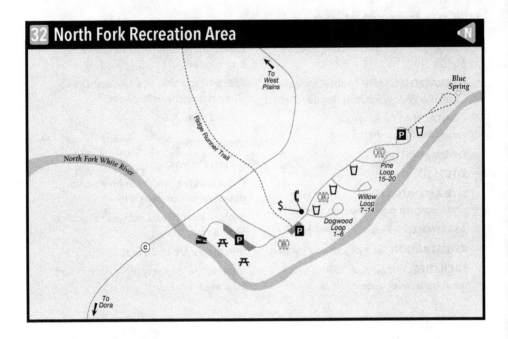

:: Getting There

From West Plains go 16 miles west on MO CC. North Fork Recreation Area is on the south side of the highway, right before MO CC crosses the North Fork of the White River.

GPS COORDINATES   N 36° 45.509'   W 92° 9.153'

33

Paddy Creek Recreation Area

Paddy Creek Recreation Area is perfect for exploring the 7,000-acre Paddy Creek Wilderness on the 17-mile Big Piney Trail.

Paddy Creek Recreation Area isn't just another nice campground—it's my favorite Missouri camping spot. I love Paddy Creek's beauty, but fun memories make it special for me too. I'll never forget waking in predawn darkness one April morning and hearing a low voice from the next site murmur, "I've got a shotgun, you've got a shotgun, he's got a shotgun . . . I guess we're ready to go." I chuckled in my sleeping bag, thankful I knew it was turkey season.

Spending a few nights at Paddy Creek might put this campground at the top of your list too. Tall bluffs overlook Paddy Creek as it curves around the campground to join the Big Piney River to the east. The campground is at the end of the road into the recreation area, so it's remote and quiet. A cooling splash in Paddy Creek is less than 200 feet from all sites. Distance between the sites is good, and all except site 23 are well shaded. Even so, I really like site 23. One tree shades its table, and an open grassy area stretches north of it. It's well suited for several tents, and its grassy

:: Ratings

BEAUTY: ★ ★ ★ ★ ★
PRIVACY: ★ ★ ★ ★ ★
SPACIOUSNESS: ★ ★ ★ ★
QUIET: ★ ★ ★ ★ ★
SECURITY: ★ ★ ★ ★
CLEANLINESS: ★ ★ ★ ★ ★

field offers a place for Frisbee, sunbathing, or stargazing. Sites 14 and 15 are the best sites at Paddy Creek, overlooking the stream at the end of the campground road.

A terrific campground for hikers, Paddy Creek is located at the eastern edge of the 7,000-acre Paddy Creek Wilderness Area. The Big Paddy and Little Paddy Creeks meander through the wilderness area. You can explore the hills and hollows around these creeks on the 17-mile Big Piney Trail. A cutoff divides this long and narrow loop into two sections, making it perfect for weekend hikers. You can hike the eastern half of the wilderness on a Saturday ramble of around 12 miles and poke around the western half on a 9-mile jaunt on Sunday. A map of Paddy Creek Wilderness is posted at the pay station in the campground, or you can print one off the Mark Twain National Forest's website. Maps and trail signs for the wilderness are confusing, referring to a South Loop and a North Loop. They really refer to the north and south sides of the Big Piney Trail. These two sides meet near Roby Lake Picnic Area, the trailhead for hiking the western half of the Big Piney Trail.

You can hike the eastern half of the Big Piney right from your campsite. Don't bother to walk to the trailhead—just cross the creek next to the camp, push about 100 feet through the woods until you strike the trail, and turn right. Just over a mile

:: Key Information

ADDRESS: 108 S. Sam Houston Blvd., Houston, MO 65483

OPERATED BY: Mark Twain NF/Houston/Rolla/Cedar Creek Ranger District

CONTACT: 417-967-4194; www.fs.usda.gov/mtnf

OPEN: Apr. 1–Dec. 1; camping permitted in picnic area Dec. 2–Mar. 31

SITES: 23

SITE AMENITIES: Table, lantern pole, fire pit with grate

ASSIGNMENT: First come, first served

REGISTRATION: Donation box at loop entrance

FACILITIES: Vault toilets, trails; no water available

PARKING: At each site

FEE: Donations accepted

ELEVATION: 890'

RESTRICTIONS:

■ **Pets:** On leash only

■ **Fires:** In fire pits; burn only wood gathered or purchased locally

■ **Alcohol:** Allowed, subject to local ordinances

■ **Vehicles:** Up to 34 feet

■ **Other:** 14-day stay limit

later you'll be enjoying an overlook of the campground and the hills to the south—a wonderful place to watch the sunset. A half mile farther is the Big Piney Trail Camp, designed for equestrians. With picnic tables in a grove of pines, it's a great place for a picnic. At 3 miles into your hike the trail crosses Forest Service Road 220. For an easy 5-mile loop, you can turn left here and follow the road back to camp.

West of FS 220 the trail enters the wilderness. About 1 mile in you'll cross a stream that's usually dry. About a quarter mile down this wash is a beautiful little box canyon and spring. Another mile past the spring is the path that cuts 1 mile across the loop to the south side of the Big Piney Trail, where a left turn heads toward the campground. The cutoff crosses Little Paddy Creek, so in spring you might get wet feet. About a half mile before reaching camp you'll get wet again, this time crossing Big Paddy Creek in a pretty bottomland just west of camp.

Don't blow off the western half of the Big Piney Trail from Roby Lake, especially in

spring, when the creeks are flowing strongly. Three miles along the south side the trail hugs several hundred yards of steep cliffs overlooking the headwaters of Little Paddy Creek. This vista faces southeast, so it's a wonderful place for a snack or napping in the morning sun. On the north side, 2.5 miles east of the trailhead, there's a rocky streambed with ledges and cascades. When the creek is flowing, an exquisite little waterfall pours off an 8-foot undercut ledge. The waterfall's undercut is so deep that you can scramble underneath and admire the wilderness through a sparkling curtain of water.

Two short trails in the area are worth a look too. The 1-mile Paddy Creek Trail starts at the picnic area and explores the creek banks to the west. Its best feature is a spectacular overlook, complete with benches and boulders for watching the sunset. The other short hike is the 2-mile Slabtown Bluff Trail at nearby Slabtown Bluff Picnic Area, a few miles to the east. It follows the Big Piney River and then climbs to a bluff overlook with incredible vistas.

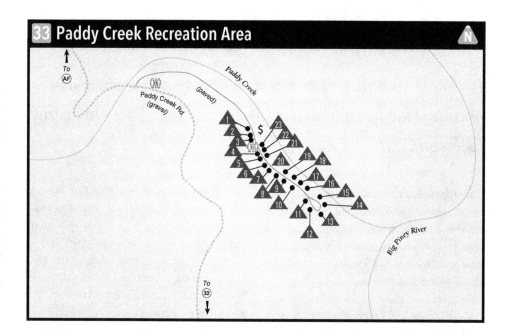

Note: To reach Roby Lake Picnic Area and the western trailhead for the Big Piney Trail, drive 1 mile north of Success, a small town west of Paddy Creek, on MO 17 to FS 274, and then go east a half mile to Roby Lake.

:: Getting There

From Licking drive 13 miles west on MO 32 to Paddy Creek Road (Forest Service Road 220). Turn right and follow this gravel road 6 miles north to Paddy Creek Recreation Area. Turn right and drive past the picnic area and trailhead to the campground at the end of the paved road.

GPS COORDINATES   N 37° 33.463'   W 92° 2.934'

34

Pine Ridge Recreation Area

Pine Ridge is a perfect hideaway for escaping the pressures of college life in Columbia or governmental silliness in nearby Jefferson City.

Pine Ridge Recreation Area is a great place to escape the hustle-bustle of college life at the University of Missouri in Columbia, or the craziness of civil service at the state capital in nearby Jefferson City. It's located in the Cedar Creek District of the Mark Twain National Forest, on land that's in the transition zone between forest and tallgrass prairie. A grove of pines planted by the Civilian Conservation Corps shades the camp, and Pine Ridge is a trailhead for the 36-mile Cedar Creek Trail. The Katy Trail, a 225-mile rails-to-trails conversion running from Clinton to St. Charles, follows the nearby Missouri River, and one of its most scenic stretches is a few miles west of Pine Ridge.

Pine Ridge reflects its name well— it's a nice hideaway in a grove of evergreens on a broad ridge. Towering pines shade every site, and a grassy open space can be used for catching rays or tossing a Frisbee. It's a very popular camp that often fills on spring and fall weekends. The recreation area is laid out in a tadpole-shaped loop

:: Ratings

BEAUTY: ★ ★ ★ ★
PRIVACY: ★ ★ ★ ★
SPACIOUSNESS: ★ ★ ★
QUIET: ★ ★ ★ ★
SECURITY: ★ ★ ★ ★
CLEANLINESS: ★ ★ ★ ★

with shady picnic sites along the entrance road. Site 1, located on the entrance road just before the loop begins, is a nice small camping spot with a cooking shelter. Site 2, located on the beginning of the loop, also has a cooking shelter and is a small camp like site 1. Sites 3 and 4 are both well spaced and private camping spots on spurs off the loop, with site 3 having the most space and good privacy. While sites 3–8 don't have cooking shelters like sites 1 and 2, they do have barbecue grills to supplement their on-the-ground fire grates.

Sites 5–8 are walk-in sites accessed from a small parking area near the beginning of the loop. Sites 6, 7, and 8 are so close to the parking lot that they're like car-camping sites. Located next to each other on lush grass shaded by tall pines, they're wonderful sites for families or small groups. You could fit several tents around each site and still have room to play Frisbee or horseshoes. Site 5 is a true walk-in site that's 50 yards across the lawn from the parking lot. It's worth the trudge, though—this secluded camping spot is the most private site at Pine Ridge Recreation Area.

The Cedar Creek Trail runs through Pine Ridge, and it's a popular ride for both equestrians and mountain bikers. It's too long a ride for many bikers, but carrying a forest map of the Cedar Creek District lets you use numerous road crossings to choose

:: Key Information

ADDRESS: 4549 MO H, Fulton, MO 65251

OPERATED BY: Mark Twain NF/Houston/Rolla/Cedar Creek Ranger District

CONTACT: 573-592-1400; www.fs.usda.gov/mtnf

OPEN: Year-round

SITES: 8

SITE AMENITIES: Table, lantern pole, fire grate; some with cooking shelter

ASSIGNMENT: First come, first served

REGISTRATION: Donation box at entrance

FACILITIES: Water, vault toilets, picnic sites, trail

PARKING: At each site

FEE: Donations accepted

ELEVATION: 780'

RESTRICTIONS:

◼ **Pets:** On leash only

◼ **Fires:** In fire pits; burn only wood gathered or purchased locally

◼ **Alcohol:** Allowed, subject to local ordinances

◼ **Vehicles:** 34 feet

◼ **Other:** 14-day stay limit; no horses allowed in Pine Ridge Recreation Area

---

loops of varying lengths for riders of differing skill and endurance levels. Where the north side of the main loop crosses Cedar Creek, you'll find Rutherford Bridge, an abandoned steel span across which a local scout troop has constructed a footbridge. Though the Cedar Creek Trail is a bit long for day hiking, a good short trek is the 4 miles from Pine Ridge to Dry Fork Recreation Area. A 1-mile hike north from Pine Ridge leads to the Nevins Homestead, two stabilized buildings from an old farmstead that's being slowly reclaimed by the forest.

Pine Ridge is a good place to camp while riding the Katy Trail. The Katy is a state park that's the longest rails-to-trails conversion in the country, stretching across two-thirds of Missouri. It was conceived in 1986, when the Missouri, Kansas, and Texas Railroad, known as the Katy, abandoned its line between Sedalia and St. Charles. The Union Pacific donated another abandoned section between Sedalia and Clinton in 1991, and in 1993, after much legal wrangling and the generous donation of $2 million by Edward "Ted" Jones, the trail was finally built. Its scenic miles along the Missouri River now draw cyclists from all over the world.

One of the best stretches of the Katy Trail, the 35-mile section between Rocheport and Jefferson City, is 15 miles west of Pine Ridge. It features limestone bluffs, old steel bridges, long stretches next to the wide Missouri River, and quaint small towns. Especially interesting is Hartsburg, a picturesque little village that serves as a trailhead for the Katy. There you'll find bike shops, bike rentals, and several restaurants. If you ride 25 miles west from Hartsburg to Rocheport, you'll see pre–Civil War houses and pedal through the only tunnel on the Katy Trail, a 243-foot-long stone arch tunnel on the west side of town.

Another spot to visit near Pine Ridge is Carrington Pits, a beautiful set of ponds formed in abandoned strip pits from an old coal-mining operation. Now filled with water and surrounded by cedars and hardwoods, these ponds are stocked with largemouth

34 Pine Ridge Recreation Area

To Ashland →

To Guthrie →

bass, sunfish, and catfish. There are picnic sites for hanging out, and a trail leads to two fishing piers on these now-scenic strip mine ponds. Carrington Pits is 3 miles west of Fulton on MO H, and then 1 mile north on County Road 315.

:: Getting There

From US 63 at Ashland, Pine Ridge Recreation Area is 7 miles east on MO Y. The campground is on the north side of the road.

GPS COORDINATES N 38° 45.471' W 92° 8.539'

35

Red Bluff Recreation Area

Admire the red bluff towering over Huzzah Creek from your campsite at the Pines Overlook.

Red Bluff Recreation Area is a forested enclave in a horseshoe bend of Huzzah Creek. The campground takes its name from the red hues in the cliff across the Huzzah. The light rusty color results from oxidization of iron compounds in the rock strata. American Indians called the bluff Painted Rock.

It seems that every streamside campground in the Ozarks was once a mill site, and Red Bluff Recreation Area is no exception. Two different mills once operated on Huzzah Creek in the 1800s. Boyer Mill, built circa 1830 near the downstream campground, was the first. Bryant's Mill followed about 30 years later, and a community named Boyer grew around the site. Over time, the community's center moved a short distance downstream and was renamed Davisville.

Though the campground is only a mile from the village of Davisville, it feels like it's in the middle of nowhere—in other words, it's a wonderful place. This streamside getaway is divided into three loops. Sites 1–23

:: Ratings

BEAUTY: ★ ★ ★ ★ ★
PRIVACY: ★ ★ ★
SPACIOUSNESS: ★ ★ ★ ★
QUIET: ★ ★ ★ ★
SECURITY: ★ ★ ★
CLEANLINESS: ★ ★ ★ ★ ★

are in the Upper Loop, where the old gristmill once operated. Though there are nice sites in this loop, it has the least shade and privacy, some sites are close together, and the ground is somewhat gravelly due to occasional flooding. The loop is very close to the creek, so if access to the stream is important to you, this is the place to be. Site 7 is closest to the Huzzah. Sites 13, 16, and 18, in shady alcoves away from the Huzzah, are the nicest sites on the Upper Loop.

Sites 24–43 are set downstream, where the Boyer Mill once stood. Scattered along a tadpole-shaped loop, these grassy spots provide better shade and spacing and are more private. Sites 24–37 are along the tadpole's tail, and you'll find electric sites 24–29 here. Sites 38–43 are on the turnaround loop at the end of the road. My favorite spot on this loop is site 30—a double site with a grassy field stretching behind it to Huzzah Creek. The group sites are just upstream from this field and are some of the best group sites in the Ozarks.

The last three sites are the prettiest camping spots at Red Bluff. A quarter mile down the entrance road, a sign on the right points to the Pines Overlook. Sites 44, 45, and 46 are in a pine grove there. Site 44 is in the woods, 100 feet from the edge of a cliff. It's a nice spot, but sites 45 and 46, the best sites in Red Bluff and quite possibly the two coolest campsites in Missouri, sit on the edge of a bluff over the wooded Huzzah Valley. With

:: Key Information

ADDRESS: 10019 West MO 8, Potosi, MO 63664

OPERATED BY: Mark Twain NF/Potosi/Fredericktown Ranger District/Monroe Campground and Recreation

CONTACT: 573-438-5427; www.fs.usda.gov/mtnf

OPEN: Mid-Apr.–mid-Oct.

SITES: 37 individual, 9 double, 3 group

SITE AMENITIES: Table, fire pit with grate, lantern pole; some with cooking shelter

ASSIGNMENT: First come, first served; reservations available at 877-444-6777 or recreation.gov

REGISTRATION: Self-pay at entrance

FACILITIES: Water, vault toilets, pavilion, picnic area, trails

PARKING: At each site; $2 day-use fee per vehicle for noncampers

FEE: $10 individual, $20 double, $17 single electric, $34 double electric, $25–$100 group; $9 nonrefundable reservation fee

ELEVATION: 800'

RESTRICTIONS:

■ **Pets:** On leash only

■ **Fires:** In fire pits; burn only wood gathered or purchased locally

■ **Alcohol:** Allowed, subject to local ordinances

■ **Vehicles:** Up to 45 feet

■ **Other:** 14-day stay limit; no glass containers in Huzzah Creek

only three sites, it won't ever be crowded at the overlook. It's always a quiet place where the only sound is the breeze sighing through the pines. If you do want to visit the main campground, it's only a short walk down the Red Bluff Trail that goes by the overlook on its way to the main campground. Unless you sleepwalk or fear heights, try for one of these three sites.

The Red Bluff Trail starts at the picnic area parking lot. It's a nice 1-mile loop through the forest above camp, past the Pines Overlook, and back to the picnic area. It's open to both hikers and mountain bikers and is suitable for novices. Another easy trail starts near the picnic area and follows the Huzzah a half mile upstream past the Red Bluff.

Huzzah Creek is the big attraction at Red Bluff Recreation Area. It has nice swimming and wading areas and is a fun tubing run through the campground. Bring your rod and reel and go after the smallmouth and rock bass lurking in the Huzzah. The Huzzah is also a fine canoe run, flowing 23 miles from the MO V bridge near the campground to the confluence with the Meramec River. It is a pretty float all the way. In dry seasons near Red Bluff, water levels may be too low, but from MO 8 to the Meramec it's usually floatable year-round. More canoeing fun is on Courtois Creek, which parallels the Huzzah a few miles to the east. The Courtois dumps into the Huzzah a bit south of the Meramec River.

Great road biking can be found on the hilly, empty highways around Davisville. The roads also allow for wonderful drives, especially during October, when fall colors peak, or in spring, when the dogwoods bloom. On your drive go to Dillard Mill State Historic Site on MO 49 and tour one of the best-preserved gristmills in the Ozarks. For mountain bikers, the Berryman Trail,

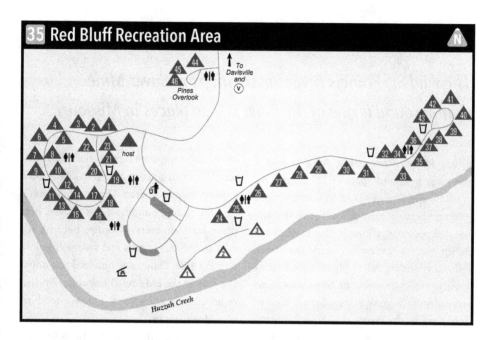

35 Red Bluff Recreation Area

thought by many to be the best ride in the state, is 15 miles to the north. Tubing, canoeing, biking, hiking, bird-watching, or just listening to the wind that whispers in the pines—there's something for everyone at Red Bluff Recreation Area.

:: Getting There

From Davisville drive 1 mile east on MO V, and then turn left into Red Bluff Recreation Area.

GPS COORDINATES   N 37° 48.428'   W 91° 10.719'

36

Silver Mines Recreation Area

The wild St. Francis River upstream from Silver Mines Campground is one of the most scenic places in Missouri.

Silver Mines Recreation Area is one of the most beautiful spots in Missouri. This is where the St. Francis River cuts a rugged canyon through granite bluffs overlooking its rocky course through the mountains. At the turn of the 20th century, the Ozark hills surrounding Silver Mines were part of a busy mining district of the forest. One reminder of those days is an old mill site and dam built by the Einstein Mining Company for processing ore for silver, lead, and other minerals. Located upstream from the bridge on MO D, the now-breached dam is one of the many rapids enjoyed by kayakers and canoeists on the St. Francis, Missouri's only whitewater river.

Now the miners are gone, their place taken by visitors to this popular recreation site in the Mark Twain National Forest. Silver Mines encompasses four campground loops, two picnic areas, a boulder-studded swimming hole, boater access sites, riverside trails, and lots of rapids and scenery.

Riverside Loop is located just south of the bridge over the St. Francis. It offers

:: Ratings

BEAUTY: ★ ★ ★ ★ ★
PRIVACY: ★ ★ ★ ★ ★
SPACIOUSNESS: ★ ★ ★ ★ ★
QUIET: ★ ★ ★ ★ ★
SECURITY: ★ ★ ★ ★
CLEANLINESS: ★ ★ ★ ★ ★

12 electric campsites next to the river, scattered on both sides of a loop road around a small grassy open area. This is where you'll find the campground host. It's also the best place for swimmers to camp, because it's next to the picnic area and swimming hole parking area. Only a few hundred feet down the road is the old MO D low-water bridge, replaced only a few years ago by a modern span downstream.

Just across the river to the north are Summit Loop, with 25 sites, and Prospect Loop, with 18 sites. Located side by side on a wooded hill above the river, they are breezier, better shaded, and offer better spacing and privacy than Riverside. They are a bit farther from the St. Francis than Riverside but are cooler and more secluded.

Spring Branch Loop is a half mile north of Prospect and Summit. Serving as overflow camping when the other three loops are full, Spring Branch's 12 sites only fill on those spring weekends when steady rains transform the St. Francis River into a whitewater paradise, attracting paddlers from all over Missouri and Arkansas. It isn't as well kept or level as the other loops, but it's built in a grove of large pine and hardwood trees that sigh in the breeze. More secluded and peaceful than the other loops, it's my favorite of the four loops at Silver Mines.

Hiking and boating are the best ways to enjoy Silver Mines. You'll need whitewater skills to run the river, though. Beginning

:: Key Information

ADDRESS: 10019 W. MO 8, Potosi, MO 63664

OPERATED BY: Mark Twain NF/Potosi/Fredericktown Ranger District/Silver Mines Campground Management

CONTACT: 573-438-5427; www.fs.usda.gov/mtnf

OPEN: Feb. 28–Oct. 30

SITES: 67 individual, 1 group

SITE AMENITIES: Table, fire pit with grate, lantern pole

ASSIGNMENT: First come, first served; reservations available at 877-444-6777 or recreation.gov

REGISTRATION: Self-pay at loop entrances

FACILITIES: Vault toilets, water spigots in each loop, picnic sites, river access, trails

PARKING: At each site; $2 day-use fee per vehicle for noncampers

FEE: $10 individual, $20 double, $17 single electric, $34 double electric; $9 nonrefundable reservation fee

ELEVATION: 600'

RESTRICTIONS:

■ **Pets:** On leash only

■ **Fires:** In fire pits; burn only wood gathered or purchased locally

■ **Alcohol:** Allowed, subject to local ordinances

■ **Vehicles:** Up to 30 feet

■ **Other:** 14-day stay limit

upstream at the MO 72 bridge, the St. Francis River challenges boaters with rapids named Land of Oz, Big Drop, Cat's Paw, Double Drop, and Rickety Rack. Each March the Missouri Whitewater Championships are held in Millstream Gardens Conservation Area, 2 miles upstream from the campgrounds.

At Millstream the river crashes through the Tiemann Shut-Ins, creating rapids that draw boaters from all over the eastern half of the United States for the races. With huge boulders in the river and a hillside sloping downward from the north side of the stream, Millstream offers an ideal setting to watch the competition and admire the spectacular rock garden in the riverbed. When graced by nice spring weather, race weekends attract as many as 2,000 spectators who relax on the boulders and enjoy picnics in the sun while watching the boaters work their way through the rapids.

If you aren't a boater, you can enjoy the river from the 2.5-mile trail that follows the St. Francis River from Silver Mines to Millstream Gardens. Along the way you'll hike through quiet forests, along high bluffs with great views, and next to the sometimes peaceful, sometimes violent St. Francis River. The hike starts at the boater's access on the north side of the river near the old MO D bridge and goes upstream. A half mile upriver is the old dam and mill site built during the area's mining days to power mining equipment. This relic is worth a look, and if the water is low, you can cross below the dam and hike back to camp on the south side of the river for a 1-mile loop. Along the way back to the campground you'll pass by an old mine shaft called Air Conditioner. Complete with a small shed and benches for relaxing, it's a perfect break on a hot summer hike. Be careful crossing the St. Francis, and don't ever attempt it if the river is flowing

36 Silver Mines Recreation Area

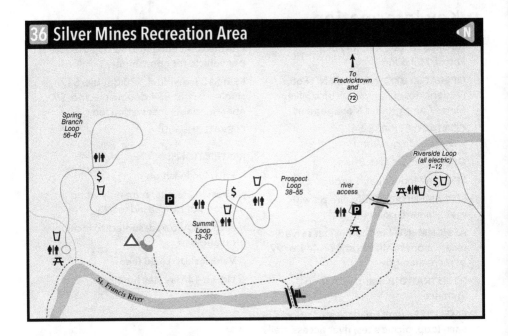

strongly. If you're uncomfortable with crossing below the dam, retrace your steps and hike up to the Air Conditioner and the dam from Riverside Loop.

Continuing upstream on the trail that follows the north riverbank, you'll pass Turkey Creek Picnic Area and then hike forests and hills for 1.5 miles until you reach Cat's Paw rapid, where a viewing platform treats you to spectacular views up and down the St.

Francis. Just beyond Cat's Paw, the river roars through the Tiemann Shut-Ins at Millstream Gardens, where you'll thump across an old wooden bridge near the picnic area at the trail's end. Though the campground is closed in winter, I love to hike this trail when it's below freezing. The bitter cold grows spectacular ice formations in the river's rapids, and once I saw an eagle perched on a limb high above the St. Francis.

:: Getting There

From Fredericktown drive 6.5 miles west on MO 72 to MO D, where you'll see a sign to Silver Mines Recreation Area. Turn left (south) on MO D and follow it 3 miles to Silver Mines. Summit, Prospect, and Spring Branch Loops are on the north side of the St. Francis River. Riverside Loop is on the south side.

To reach Millstream Gardens, drive 8 miles west of Fredericktown on MO 72, turn south at the wooden sign for Millstream Gardens, and follow a gravel road 0.5 mile to the parking area.

GPS COORDINATES   N 37° 33.285'   W 90° 26.026'

37

Sutton Bluff Recreation Area

Hike the Sutton Bluff Trail for scenic views over a horseshoe bend in the Black River.

Sutton Bluff Recreation Area is named for R. G. Sutton, who settled this valley on the Black River in 1888. Three generations of Suttons farmed the river bottoms below the impressive bluff just upstream from the campground. A pretty meander of the Black River curls around the campsites, and another wooded bluff rises steeply to the west to shade the campground in the late afternoon. Sutton Bluff is a wonderful place for hiking, picnicking, mountain biking, canoeing, swimming, or just hanging out.

Newly renovated after the 2009 windstorm that devastated forests all over southern Missouri, Sutton Bluff's campground features a newly paved loop road and parking spurs. Just enough trees survived the storm to shade most sites. While electricity has been added to 14 sites in the northern half of the campground, the loop's southern half remains comfortably primitive. All camping spots here are good ones, but the best sites are 7, 9, 11, 13, and 14. These are single sites on the southern part of the loop, only a few steps from the river. Site 14 is the

:: Ratings

BEAUTY: ★ ★ ★ ★ ★
PRIVACY: ★ ★ ★
SPACIOUSNESS: ★ ★ ★ ★
QUIET: ★ ★ ★
SECURITY: ★ ★ ★ ★
CLEANLINESS: ★ ★ ★ ★ ★

best of all—it's the most private spot in the campground. Site 15, a secluded spot next to the river, is Sutton's group camp. Sites 16–34 are on the gentle hillside sloping upward from the river. Most have level spots for tents, and those at the far end of the camp are quiet with a view of the rest of the campground. Water and restrooms are scattered conveniently throughout the campground.

If the campground is full or you just want to really go primitive (and cheap), check out Sutton Bluff's free campsites. They're across the river on the west side of the road, where several picnic tables and fire rings are scattered around a small meadow. No toilets or water are available here, but you'll be right across the gravel bar from the campground's namesake bluff—a really nice spot for wading, swimming, or sunbathing. You can use facilities in the developed part of camp, but expect the campground host to charge you a $2 day-use fee.

The river attracts many campers. You can fish right from the campground, hiking up- or downstream to try your luck. The river bend that wraps around the campground is only a few steps away, and it's a great place to swim, wade, or relax in the sun with your lawn chair and a cold drink. Just upstream from camp, Forest Service Road 2236 crosses the river bridge. The broad gravel bar above the bridge, overlooked by Sutton Bluff, is a wonderful place to play in the water or watch the sunset. The

:: Key Information

ADDRESS: 1301 S. Main St., Salem, MO 65560

OPERATED BY: Mark Twain NF/Salem Ranger District

CONTACT: 573-729-6656; www.fs.usda.gov/mtnf

OPEN: Late Mar.–early Nov.

SITES: 26 individual, 6 double, 1 group

SITE AMENITIES: Table, fire pit with grate, lantern pole

ASSIGNMENT: First come, first served; reservations available at 877-444-6777 or recreation.gov

REGISTRATION: Self-pay at entrance or host will collect

FACILITIES: Water, flush and vault toilets, showers, pavilion, picnic sites, trails, horseshoe pits, phone

PARKING: At each site; $2 day-use fee per vehicle for noncampers

FEE: $8 single, $15 single electric, $16 double, $25 double electric, $40 group camp; $34 pavilion; $9 nonrefundable reservation fee

ELEVATION: 820'

RESTRICTIONS:

■ **Pets:** On leash only

■ **Fires:** In fire pits; burn only wood gathered or purchased locally

■ **Alcohol:** Allowed, subject to local ordinances

■ **Vehicles:** Up to 60 feet

■ **Other:** 14-day stay limit; no glass containers in river

Black River is great for tubing and canoeing, and outfitters in nearby Lesterville can equip you for a relaxing float through the forested mountains.

There are two places to mountain bike right from camp. One of these is the Sutton Bluff ATV Trails, a series of point-to-point routes of various lengths. Using forest roads as connectors, on the trail system you can ride loops of 3–10 miles. They're scattered along FS 2233 and are marked with orange posts and numbers. The campground host usually has maps of the Sutton Bluff ATV Trails, or you can contact the U.S. Forest Service in Salem.

The other bike ride follows the Karkaghne section of the Ozark Trail. I always wondered where this strange name came from, and the folks at the Mark Twain National Forest finally gave me the straight scoop. Karkaghne is named for a mystical, dragonlike forest creature that usually walks backward. It doesn't much care

where it's going, but it likes to know where it's been. Only a few lucky individuals have seen this shy, secretive beast, usually through the bottom of a fruit jar recently emptied of moonshine. Well, that's what they told me.

Anyway, the Karkaghne Trail is tough but nice. It runs 18 miles west from Sutton Bluff to the junction of MO 72 and MO P, and 10 miles north to Oates on MO J. Going west, the first part of the Karkaghne section is very rugged and has several long climbs, but once past mile 6 it's a good ride all the way to the trailhead at MO 72. You can make a 30-mile loop by biking the trail to MO 72, and then returning to Sutton Bluff via MO 72, MO TT, County Road 854, and FS 2236. The Karkaghne Trail leaves Sutton Bluff from the far end of the concrete bridge, heading uphill to the west.

The most scenic part of the Karkaghne section of the Ozark Trail is right next to the camp. You can hike this path on the 2-mile

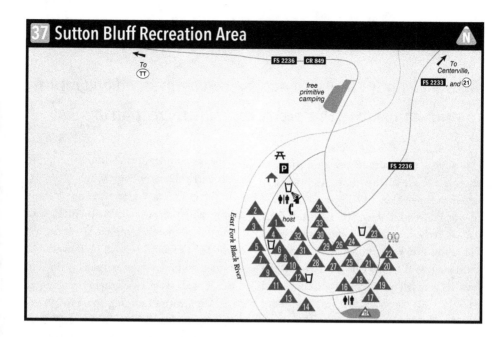

37 Sutton Bluff Recreation Area

Sutton Bluff Trail. Following the Karkaghne for its first mile, the trail switchbacks steeply up the northern end of the bluff overlooking the camp. Once near the top, it cuts straight across the cliff face, with beautiful overlooks and drop-offs steep enough to require handrails. Along the highest part of the hike you'll enjoy dramatic views of the Black River's horseshoe bend around the campground. Soon after the path leaves the cliff edge, you'll come to a fork. The Sutton Bluff Trail follows the left fork, descends to the Black

River, and follows the riverbank back to the trailhead. This is an especially great hike in the fall, when the colors are blazing, and it's pretty nice in winter, when less foliage makes for even more spectacular views. It can be a hot trudge in summer, but thoughts of a dip in the river at the trail's end will keep you stepping happily along.

While you're at Sutton Bluff, keep an eye peeled for those Karkaghnes. Because fruit jars aren't allowed in the river, you probably won't see any.

:: Getting There

From Centerville drive north 3 miles on MO 21 to Forest Service Road 2233, where a sign directs you to Sutton Bluff. Turn left and go 7 miles to FS 2236/County Road 849, where another sign directs you left 3 miles to the campground.

GPS COORDINATES   N 37° 28.651'   W 91° 0.374' 39

38

Watercress Recreation Area

Take a leisurely stroll to a nearby ice-cream stand and return to your campsite in this pretty riverside recreation area.

Have you ever dreamed of slurping a chocolate shake while you were camping out under the open skies? Well, you can do just that at Watercress Recreation Area. It feels like it's in the middle of nowhere, yet it's less than a mile from downtown Van Buren. It's a short walk to the Jolly Cone, where you can founder yourself on ice cream and then head back to your campsite to complain about how much you ate.

Watercress Recreation Area is next to the Current River, on a small flatland between the stream and the hills that separate the campground from Van Buren. The campground at Watercress was completely remodeled around 2010, and unlike other campground upgrades I've seen, this one is better for it. They did lay too much asphalt and spread too much gravel, but most sites are roomier than before and have nicer areas to pitch your tent. Six sites are accessible. Cold-water outdoor showers were added to the day-use area, so you can clean and cool yourself on those hot and humid Missouri summer days, and pavilions allow you to

ride out a thunderstorm without having to hole up in a claustrophobic tent.

The 17 sites at Watercress line up along a long and narrow loop, with most sites being fairly roomy camping spots on the outside of the loop. A small bluff overlooks the first part of the loop, and sites 3, 5, 6, and 9 nestle against the creek that runs along its base. My favorite camping spots in Watercress are 13–17 at the end of the loop. Sites 13–15 are shady alcoves in the woods, and you can see the Current River from 15. Sites 16 and 17 are right on the river's edge. With nice space for your tent, site 16 is the better of these two. Site 17 is good, but you'll have to pitch your tent on gravel if you camp in this spot. It would be a great site for a camper van or pop-up.

The Current River is the immediate attraction at this campground. It's wide and slow as it passes Watercress Spring, an ideal spot for tubing, swimming, wading, and fishing from the riverbanks. At one time this broad, shallow reach of the Current was used as a ford. During the Civil War, 3,000 Union troops camped here, with a mission of suppressing guerilla warfare in the surrounding countryside. They built breastworks on the hills above the current campground site and kept a close eye on the river crossing for Confederate operations.

You can examine the remains of their encampment from the 1.2-mile Songbird Trail. Beginning at the spring, this hike

:: Ratings

BEAUTY: ★ ★ ★ ★
PRIVACY: ★ ★ ★
SPACIOUSNESS: ★ ★ ★
QUIET: ★ ★ ★ ★
SECURITY: ★ ★ ★ ★ ★
CLEANLINESS: ★ ★ ★ ★ ★

:: Key Information

ADDRESS: MO 19 N., Winona, MO 65588

OPERATED BY: Mark Twain NF/Eleven Point Ranger District

CONTACT: 573-325-4233; www.fs.usda.gov/mtnf

OPEN: Late Apr.-Oct. 31

SITES: 15 individual, 2 double

SITE AMENITIES: Table, fire pit with grate, lantern pole; many with cooking shelter

ASSIGNMENT: First come, first served

REGISTRATION: Self-pay station at loop entrance

FACILITIES: Water, flush and vault toilets, cold showers in day-use area, pavilions, picnic area, river access

PARKING: At each site

FEE: $10 single, $15 double; $25 pavilion

ELEVATION: 460'

RESTRICTIONS:

■ **Pets:** On leash only

■ **Fires:** In fire pits; burn only wood gathered or purchased locally

■ **Alcohol:** Allowed, subject to local ordinances

■ **Vehicles:** Up to 40 feet

■ **Other:** 14-day stay limit; 8-person limit per site (16 for doubles); no glass containers in river or on its banks

follows the spring branch and climbs onto the hill above camp. From the ridge near the headquarters building you'll see the soldiers' old trenches on the slope below the trail. A plaque tells the legend of an old cannon that had to be left behind when the troops moved out. To keep it out of Confederate hands, the Union troops supposedly shoved it off the hillside into the spring branch flowing through camp. If the myth is true, the cannon is still buried in the silt under the calm spring creek at Watercress.

My favorite attraction in the area is the Ozark National Scenic Riverways' Big Spring, located 5 miles south of Watercress on MO 103. You can camp there, but I prefer camping at the more laid-back Watercress Recreation Area and driving over to Big Spring to admire that area's beauty as a day user, picking up an ice cream cone or a cheeseburger as I cruise through downtown Van Buren.

Big Spring truly lives up to its name—it's the biggest spring in Missouri. Flowing 286

million gallons per day, it's an aquamarine wonder. Dye tracings show that this huge gusher draws water from a 1,000-square-mile area, pulling runoff from as far away as 40 miles. After admiring the spring, you can explore the area on the Chubb Hollow Trail and the Slough Trail. These short hikes take you through the bottoms along the spring branch, past the confluence of the branch and the Current River, and over the wooded ridges above Big Spring.

The architecture of the park's lodge and cabins is worth checking out. Civilian Conservation Corps Companies 734, 1710, and 1740 built them in the 1930s as part of what was then Big Spring State Park. The National Park Service has restored these old structures. The rustic lodge, built next to the confluence of Big Spring's outflow branch and the Current River, is a wonderful place to enjoy a relaxing meal while you admire the streams flowing together outside your window. Interpretive displays in

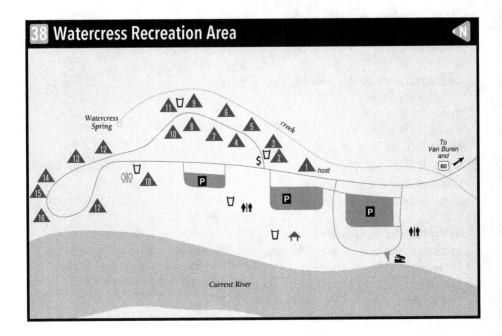

38 Watercress Recreation Area

the park describe the area's historic CCC days. To learn more about Big Spring, see the profile on page 59.

You can rent a canoe from one of several outfitters in Van Buren and float the Current down to Big Spring. It's only a 5-mile paddle from Watercress down to Big Spring, so you'll have plenty of time to explore the area after drifting down from Watercress. Bring your rod and reel—the Current has nice populations of bass, sunfish, and catfish on its run past Watercress Spring.

:: Getting There

From Van Buren's town center, go east on US 60 Business to Watercress Road. There you'll see a sign directing you to the Ozark National Scenic Riverways Headquarters and Visitor Center. Turn north, and drive a quarter mile to the visitor center. On your left across from the visitor center, you'll see the entrance to Watercress Recreation Area. Follow the blacktop road down the hill to the campground.

GPS COORDINATES   N 37° 0.022'   W 91° 0.997'

Buffalo National River

39

Kyle's Landing

To see the best of the Buffalo, float the river 10 miles from Ponca to Kyle's and spend the next day hiking the Ponca Wilderness.

Kyle's Landing is my favorite campground on the Buffalo National River. A low bluff overlooks Kyle's, and a large pine grove in the downstream end of camp reminds me of the Rockies. The campground's rough, steep 3-mile entrance road keeps RVs and monster trailers away—in fact, a sign at the campground turnoff on AR 74 recommends that you have a high-clearance, four-wheel drive vehicle. I've made the trip numerous times in my front-wheel drive Mazda 626, though, so unless it has rained recently, you should have no problem in smaller vehicles. Level grassy areas make it seem like you're camping in your backyard rather than in incredibly rugged and scenic parklands. The trails leading from Kyle's are perfect avenues for exploring those towering hills and deep hollows.

As you enter Kyle's and intersect the campground's loop road, the pine grove is on your right. Sites 1–10, scattered among these trees, are the best-shaded spots. Sites 5 and 6 are the most private, tucked far back in the evergreens. The loop then curves past the river access and sites 11–16 on an open lawn next to the river. Sites 17–19, nestled in a little meadow in the woods next to the Buffalo, are great camping spots. With good shade, privacy, and a swimming hole in the Buffalo a few feet away, they're the best sites for those who love solitude and camping next to water. Sites 20–24 are spacious and in the center of the campground loop, but they have little shade and are near the bathrooms and their all-night lights. The remaining sites are against the woods at the edge of the campground. All sites are walk-in.

Avoid Kyle's on spring weekends, especially Memorial Day and Easter, when floatable river levels attract hundreds of canoeists to the upper river. By midsummer the hordes move downriver, and Kyle's becomes a peaceful place. Fall attracts quite a few hikers, but they aren't as many or as rowdy as the spring canoeing parties. I like winter at Kyle's—days are often sunny and warm, low river levels make easy river fords on hikes from the campground, winter's lack of foliage opens up wonderful vistas along the river, and there are no camping fees.

The trailhead lies at the campground's western end. Bring the Trails Illustrated map *Buffalo River–West Half* to help you find your way on the many hiking choices from Kyle's. You can choose between the Old River Trail that stays low along the river, the Buffalo

:: Ratings

BEAUTY: ★ ★ ★ ★ ★
PRIVACY: ★ ★ ★
SPACIOUSNESS: ★ ★ ★ ★ ★
QUIET: ★ ★ ★ ★
SECURITY: ★ ★ ★ ★
CLEANLINESS: ★ ★ ★ ★ ★

:: Key Information

ADDRESS: 402 N. Walnut, Ste. 136, Harrison, AR 72601

OPERATED BY: National Park Service

CONTACT: 870-365-2700; nps.gov/buff

OPEN: Year-round

SITES: 33 walk-in

SITE AMENITIES: Table, fire pit with grate, lantern pole

ASSIGNMENT: First come, first served

REGISTRATION: At pay station next to restrooms

FACILITIES: Apr.-Oct.: Water, flush toilets; Year-round: Vault toilets, river access, trails

PARKING: At lots near sites

FEE: Mid-Mar.–mid-Nov.: $10; Mid-Nov.–mid-Mar.: free

ELEVATION: 900'

RESTRICTIONS:

■ **Pets:** On 6-foot leash at campground; not allowed on trails

■ **Fires:** In fire pits; burn only wood gathered or purchased locally

■ **Alcohol:** Allowed, subject to Arkansas state laws

■ **Vehicles:** No length limit; high-clearance four-wheel drive advised; RVs and trailers not recommended

■ **Other:** 14-day stay limit; 6-person limit per site; no glass containers in the river, in caves, on trails, or within 100 feet of any stream

River Trail that explores the highlands to the river's south, or the fantastic scramble up Indian Creek. When the river is waist-deep or less, I like the Old River Trail, a level 2 miles and four river crossings from Kyle's west to Horseshoe Bend. The trail passes two old homesteads on the way, including one with an intact barn near a lonesome old stone chimney in the overgrowth. Horseshoe Bend has a wide rock bench above the river that's a great place for a picnic, backpack camping, or hanging out.

From Horseshoe Bend it's a 1-mile hike across the river north to Hemmed-In Hollow. Hemmed-In is a monstrous box canyon with a 175-foot waterfall pouring off the bluff and showering the canyon floor below. This place is spectacular in spring or after rain, when the falls are running wild. On your return, go right at the fork you passed on the way in. Follow it a half mile uphill to a trail junction. From the junction, a quarter-mile hike uphill to the right leads to California

Point and a vista of Hemmed-In Hollow. Check out the view; then take the left trail. It follows a benchland with great views of the river, and then drops back to river level at Sneed's Creek, where you'll hit the Old River Trail. Just to your left will be the ruins of the Center Point School—I'd have loved to go to school there.

Horseshoe Bend and the route back to Kyle's is a quarter mile to the left on the Old River Trail. For more spectacular scenery, go right instead, following signs to the Center Point Trailhead. A half mile from Sneed's Creek is Granny Henderson's Cabin, an old farmhouse with a wonderful view from the front porch. From Granny's follow the Center Point Trail a mile uphill to another trail going left. This is the Goat Trail onto Big Bluff. It will take you onto a narrow ledge 350 feet above the river for the best view in all of Arkansas. Be very careful out there—it's a long fall to the river. From Big Bluff it's 4 miles back to Kyle's.

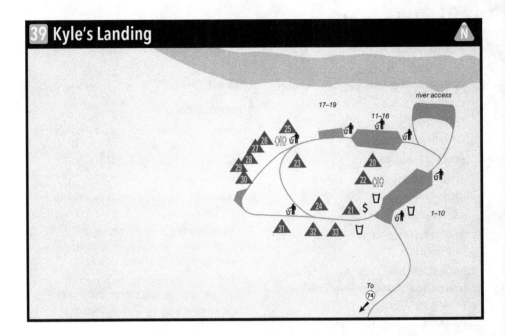

39 Kyle's Landing

While you're at Kyle's, don't miss Indian Creek, a primitive unmarked route breaking south off the Buffalo River Trail just west of camp. It's wonderful in spring or after rainstorms, when water brings this hidden canyon to life. The trail is an unbelievable succession of waterfalls, pools, cascades, bluffs, and boulders. It features a cave with a waterfall gurgling from its mouth, with another cascade rushing down a 50-foot bluff behind it. If you climb the steep hillside opposite the cave, ease through a natural tunnel in the rock and hike another quarter mile up-canyon to see a natural bridge called Eye of the Needle. Plan to spend all day in this magical canyon.

:: Getting There

Take AR 74 5 miles west from Jasper or 10 miles east from Ponca. Turn north at the sign for Kyle's Landing and follow a steep, crooked, and rough gravel road 3 miles to the campground.

GPS COORDINATES   N 36° 3.326'   W 93° 16.827'

40

Ozark

Ozark is near the Erbie Trails, where you can check out many fascinating historic sites.

Ozark doesn't have the grand bluffs found at Steel Creek, but this peaceful riverside hideaway is a comfortable place to relax. Its campsites form a ring around a grassy meadow next to the Buffalo River. The campground has both open and shaded sites, access to good day floats upstream and downstream, and a pavilion for escaping hot sunshine or chilly rainstorms.

All of these walk-in sites are level, and most are spacious. Sites 1–6 are shaded, but they're close to the loop road and far from the river. Sites 7–14 are on a bench below the level of the rest of the campground. They're farthest from the road, requiring the longest walk, but surrounding grassy expanses make them good for small groups. Sites 15–20, nestled against the fringe of trees next to the Buffalo, are closest to the river and not far from their parking spots. Sites 21–31 are the best sites at Ozark. Though they're farther from parking than other sites, these are the most private sites in the camp and are only a few steps from the river.

Ozark is an excellent canoe camp. It's a 9-mile float downstream to Hasty, easily done in a day. Upstream, you can take a nice 12-mile float from Kyle's Landing or a shorter 6-mile paddle from Erbie back to Ozark, drifting beneath impressive bluffs that tower above the river. You'll find outfitters in nearby Jasper, along with a nice selection of restaurants and shops.

The Buffalo River Trail passes Ozark, giving you hiking options right from your campsite. A 2.5-mile hike east takes you to Pruitt, the eastern terminus to this section of the trail. A 1.7-mile hike upstream goes to the Cedar Grove Overlook, where you will discover a nice view of the river and a spur trail that leads to a picnic area. While you're hiking keep an eye out for elk—they're common in this part of the Buffalo National River. I once hiked into a group of 18 of these huge critters on the Farmer Trail.

For more great hiking, go to Erbie, 1 mile south of Ozark turnoff on AR 7 and then 6 miles northwest on a gravel county road. There's a campground at Erbie, but it was closed in 2013 due to the sequester. Too bad—it's a nice place, and there are several good trails and historic sites near the camp—but you can easily explore them from Ozark Campground. The trailhead for these hikes is 2 miles beyond Erbie Campground.

One of these historic sites is the Parker-Hickman Farmstead, a half mile beyond Erbie Campground on your way to the Erbie Church trailhead. Built in the 1840s and occupied until 1977, the farm consists of a

:: Ratings

BEAUTY: ★ ★ ★ ★
PRIVACY: ★ ★ ★
SPACIOUSNESS: ★ ★ ★ ★
QUIET: ★ ★ ★ ★
SECURITY: ★ ★ ★ ★ ★
CLEANLINESS: ★ ★ ★ ★ ★

:: Key Information

ADDRESS: 402 N. Walnut, Ste. 136, Harrison, AR 72601

OPERATED BY: National Park Service

CONTACT: 870-365-2700; nps.gov/buff

OPEN: Year-round

SITES: 31 walk-in sites

SITE AMENITIES: Table, lantern pole, fire pit with grate

ASSIGNMENT: First come, first served

REGISTRATION: At self-pay station near loop entrance

FACILITIES: Mid-Mar.–mid-Nov.: Water; Year-round: Flush toilets, pavilion, river access, trails

PARKING: In lots near sites

FEE: Mid-Mar.–mid-Nov.: $10; Mid-Nov.–mid-Mar.: free

ELEVATION: 810'

RESTRICTIONS:

■ **Pets:** On 6-foot leash; not allowed on trails

■ **Fires:** In fire pits; burn only wood gathered or purchased locally

■ **Alcohol:** Allowed, subject to Arkansas state laws

■ **Vehicles:** No length limit

■ **Other:** 14-day stay limit; 6-person limit per site; no glass containers in the river, in caves, on trails, or within 100 feet of any stream

house, two barns, a chicken coop, and several other outbuildings. You can walk through the site, check out the buildings, and imagine old days on the Buffalo. I especially liked the decades-old wallpaper backing in these old rooms—newspapers with articles from times past, outdated ads such as the one reading "Fits Cured," and faded sheet music for "My Gretchen" adorn one living room wall.

You can begin your hike directly from the homestead—the Buffalo River Trail goes right through it. The best trailhead is near another historic site, the Erbie Church. It was built in 1896 and is still being used for occasional services to this day. To reach it, continue northwest from the Parker-Hickman site, splash through the river on a slab bridge, and drive a half mile to a trailhead just past the old church. The church is always unlocked, so you can check out this peaceful house of worship before you hit the trail.

Several trails take off from this trailhead, but my favorite is the Cecil Cove Loop. It uses parts of the Cecil Cove and Farmer Trails for a 7.5-mile hike. Along Cecil Creek you'll see a spring and an impressive wall built from rocks cleared from long-disappeared farm fields. You'll cross the creek several times and pass by the mouth of Beauty Cave, the longest cave in Arkansas.

The loop's southern half climbs to a ridge above Cecil Creek, passes several abandoned homesites with overgrown chimneys and daffodils and irises in season, and goes by the haunting Jones Cemetery. Several tombstones for day-old infants will make you realize how tough times were in the early 1900s on the Buffalo. Near the end of the loop you can explore the J. W. Farmer homestead, with its old house, two barns, and several outbuildings. The last leg of the hike goes past scenic Goat Bluff and an overlook of the Buffalo River. When you get back to the trailhead, the picnic table there is a wonderful place for a well-deserved posthike snack.

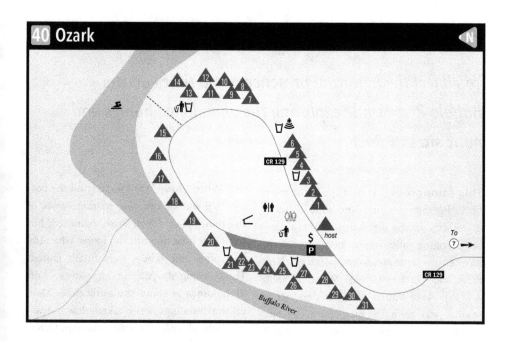

:: Getting There

From Jasper drive 4.5 miles north on AR 7 to a gravel road with a sign directing you to Ozark. Turn left and follow the gravel road 1.5 miles to the campground.

GPS COORDINATES   N 36° 3.795'   W 93° 9.644'

41

Rush

You'll feel the haunting presence of old times on the Buffalo River while exploring the abandoned homes and mine sites at Rush.

This campground is near the ghost town of Rush, "the town that zinc built." Discovery of zinc in the 1880s turned this sleepy little farming valley into a noisy boomtown. At one time, 17 mines were operating along Rush and Clabber Creeks. When in 1886 a faulty assay hinted of silver deposits, a smelter was built for processing the ore. No silver was found, but the smelter still stands in the old Morning Star Mining Company's abandoned mill complex.

Activity in the Rush Mining District reached its peak during World War I, when zinc prices jumped. Around 5,000 people lived and worked along Rush Creek in a community stretching from the present-day ghost town all the way to the Buffalo River. The end of the district near the Buffalo was called New Town, while the northern end, where old buildings still remain, was the village of Rush. Besides residences and mines, the banks of Rush Creek once held hotels, stores, a livery stable, a post office, a doctor's office, and a school.

:: Ratings

BEAUTY: ★ ★ ★ ★
PRIVACY: ★ ★
SPACIOUSNESS: ★ ★ ★ ★ ★
QUIET: ★ ★ ★
SECURITY: ★ ★ ★
CLEANLINESS: ★ ★ ★ ★ ★

When World War I ended and the bottom fell out of the zinc market, most of the mines shut down. Rush dwindled, but somehow held on until the 1960s, when the post office and school were finally closed. The Morning Star Mining Company sold off its holdings at about the same time. Most of the buildings were taken down, leaving behind only the haunting structures, scattered foundations, and mine shafts to evoke memories of the wild times in Rush and New Town. As you explore this narrow, quiet valley, you'll have a hard time believing 5,000 souls once inhabited the place.

Where Rush Creek trickles into the Buffalo River, New Town once teemed with activity. Now you can camp the peaceful riverside where the village once stood. This campground is an appealing place to hang out. It has a river to swim, fish to catch, trails to hike, and a ghost town to explore. The walk-in campground has 12 spacious, widely scattered campsites nestled in a bend of the Buffalo River. Sites 1–6 are in a long and narrow open space stretching from the campground to the river. These wooded sites have the best shade at Rush but are very sandy and have little grass.

Rush's other six sites are scattered across a small grassy field southeast of the toilets. Sites 7–10 are set against riverside trees on the east side of the field, with overhanging trees shading them until late afternoon. Sites

:: Key Information

ADDRESS: 402 N. Walnut St.,
Ste. 136, Harrison, AR 72601

OPERATED BY: National Park Service

CONTACT: 870-365-2700; nps.gov/buff

OPEN: Early spring–late fall; dates vary
from season to season. Rush may open
year-round in future years.

SITES: 12 walk-in

EACH SITE HAS: Table, fire pit with
grate, lantern pole

ASSIGNMENT: First come, first served

REGISTRATION: At pay station next to
vault toilets

FACILITIES: Water, vault toilets

PARKING: In adjacent lot

FEE: $10

ELEVATION: 475'

RESTRICTIONS:

▪ **Pets:** On 6-foot leash at campground;
not allowed on trails

▪ **Fires:** In fire pits

▪ **Alcohol:** Allowed, subject to Arkansas
state laws

▪ **Vehicles:** No length limit, but no room
for trailers or RVs at walk-in sites

▪ **Other:** 14-day stay limit; no glass containers on trails, in river, or within 50 feet
of streams; do not enter abandoned
mine shafts

11 and 12 are uphill from the river, but both are nice places to pitch your tent. Site 11 is shaded by a cedar tree and the woods along the south edge of the meadow, and a small grove of trees shelters site 12.

All sites in the field would be great sites for winter camping, but that was no longer an option when this book went to press. Rush was closed by the 2013 sequester, but a group of local residents and businesses who love the place struck a deal with the National Park Service to assist in its care and operation to reopen the campground. In the future, perhaps Rush may once again be open year-round, but as of fall 2013 the camp was open only from spring to late fall. Dates of operation may vary from year to year, so check with the NPS when planning a campout at Rush, especially near the beginning or end of the season, to make sure it's open.

Across Rush Creek from the camp are the river landing, picnic shelter, swimming hole, and trailhead. Spring, when most floaters are on the more exciting upper Buffalo, is a nice time to come to Rush. Summer, when the upper river is no longer floatable and the crowds flock to the lower part of the Buffalo, is busiest. I love to camp here in late fall and winter, when there's water in the river and nobody around except the wandering ghosts of New Town and Rush.

Trailheads are at the river access near the campground and at the Morning Star mill site near the ghost town. The 1.6-mile Rush Mountain Trail connects the river access and the campground to the abandoned Morning Star Mining Company's mill complex. Along the path you'll pass lots of old mine shafts, tailings piles, and an abandoned mine car used for hauling ore out of the earth. From the river access, a spur off this trail leads to the old Monte Cristo Mine and the Clabber Creek Overlook. From Monte Cristo an unofficial trail leads back to the Morning Star Trailhead, but it's rough and unmarked.

The Morning Star Trail is a 0.3-mile loop through the old Morning Star mill

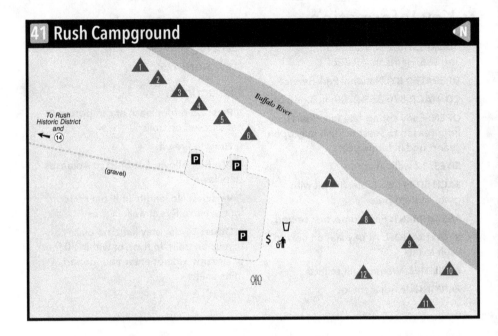

41 Rush Campground

site. It passes the remains of the blacksmith shop, foundations of the old mill building, and the still-intact 1886 smelter. A sad stop on this loop is a photo and interpretive display of the Morning Star Barn. The barn stood intact on this site from the 1890s until December 1998, when it and the nearby Brantley house were burned to the ground by arsonists.

A free guide for the Rush Mountain Trail is available at the Buffalo Point Information Station not far from Rush. While you're there, pick up a guide for the 3.5-mile Indian Rockhouse Trail at Buffalo Point and take this wonderful interpretive hike. It showcases a bluff cave that once sheltered American Indians, in addition to many Ozark natural features. The Indian Rockhouse Trailhead is near Buffalo Point's bluff-top restaurant, where you can enjoy some posthike snacking and admire the river valley hundreds of feet below your table.

:: Getting There

From Yellville, drive 11.5 miles southeast on AR 14 to the marked road to Rush. Turn left and follow this paved road to a T-intersection with a gravel road. Turn right and enter the Rush District. The camping area is 1.5 miles down on the right.

GPS COORDINATES   N 36° 7.382'   W 92° 33.018'

42

Steel Creek

Steel Creek showcases the huge stone bluffs towering above the upper Buffalo River.

Steel Creek Campground is in a grassy bottomland tucked into a wide bend of the Buffalo River. You'll often spot elk in the open grasslands between the river access and the campground. Though its openness limits privacy, the place pays you back with wonderful views of the mile-long valley. Roark Bluff dominates the skyline to the north, overlooking the valley for most of its length. Heavy downpours in Steel Creek awaken the splendid waterfalls that cascade off Roark Bluff. One of the falls forms a curtain of whitewater rolling over the bluff edge. My favorite waterfall jets off the bluff across from camp and arches almost all the way across the river.

All sites at Steel Creek are walk-in, but because the campground is a long and narrow stretch of open lawn along the river, with parking along its entire length, it's not a long slog to any site. Take the extra effort to schlep your stuff to the far side of the campground, though—you'll get away from the dust of the gravel parking lot and will be in one of the 12 sites tucked into the riverbank trees, where

there is shade and more privacy. The best spot is site 26 at the far end of the campground.

Steel Creek is very crowded in spring, when the upper river is in prime floating condition. If you like quiet, don't even consider coming here on Easter and Memorial Day weekends. Off-season is great—I once spent a rainy Thanksgiving weekend here, sharing the camp with a smattering of fellow campers and enjoying rare off-season floatable river levels. Once spring is past and the river levels drop, Steel Creek is a relaxing place to be. There's usually just enough water left in the river's pools for a cooling dip to offset summer heat, and the canoeing hordes are gone.

After canoeing, hiking is the prime activity at Steel Creek. Both Buffalo River and Old River Trails pass through the campground, giving you one upstream and two downstream hiking options. My favorite is the 2-mile hike on the Buffalo River Trail from Steel Creek to Ponca. It climbs out of camp up to Bee Bluff and follows its rim for a while. The bluff is named for a bee colony that lived high in the bluff for decades before settlers finally figured out how to get at the honey 80 feet above their heads. The trail passes a tall pillar leaning away from the bluff—close enough that you'll be tempted to jump out to it, but just far enough that you won't. Going farther on the trail will take you through a gap between the bluff and a slice of rock that has leaned away.

:: Ratings

BEAUTY: ★ ★ ★ ★ ★
PRIVACY: ★ ★
SPACIOUSNESS: ★ ★ ★ ★ ★
QUIET: ★ ★ ★ ★
SECURITY: ★ ★ ★ ★
CLEANLINESS: ★ ★ ★ ★ ★

:: Key Information

ADDRESS: 402 N. Walnut, Ste. 136, Harrison, AR 72601

OPERATED BY: National Park Service

CONTACT: 870-365-2700; nps.gov/buff

OPEN: Year-round

SITES: 26 walk-in, 14 at horse camp

SITE AMENITIES: Table, fire pit with grate, lantern pole

ASSIGNMENT: First come, first served

REGISTRATION: At pay station near toilets for walk-ins; at fork in entrance road for horse camp

FACILITIES: Mid-Mar.–mid-Nov.: Water, flush toilets; Year-round: Vault toilets, phone, trails, river access

PARKING: Lot south of walk-in campsites

FEE: Mid-Mar.–mid-Nov.: $10; Mid-Nov.–mid-Mar.: free

ELEVATION: 1,000'

RESTRICTIONS:

■ **Pets:** On 6-foot leash at campground; not allowed on trails

■ **Fires:** In fire pits; burn only wood gathered or purchased locally

■ **Alcohol:** Allowed, subject to Arkansas state laws

■ **Vehicles:** No length limit; only equestrian sites suitable for RVs and trailers

■ **Other:** 14-day stay limit; 6-person limit per site; no glass containers in river, in caves, on trails, or within 100 feet of streams

The last mile to Ponca is best. During and after rainstorms several waterfalls cascade down the hillside and splash into the Buffalo. At one point two waterfalls come snaking down the hillside, join forces near the trail, and then continue downhill as a single roaring stream. At another cascade a quarter mile from Ponca, the stream rushes over a slickrock streambed for 100 feet, and then plunges off a 50-foot bluff into the river. Just past this cascade is a stretch of trail on a bluff edge with nice views of the Buffalo.

The Buffalo River Trail east from camp is another great hike. In the first mile you'll walk over some tall rock ledges that sport a nice waterfall during wet times. When you cross Steel Creek and start climbing, you'll be in the Ponca Wilderness—one of the most beautiful landscapes in Arkansas. Just 1.5 miles from camp is the Steel Creek Overlook, one of the more scenic views in the park. On the outside of a sharp bend in the river, this cliff overlook surveys all the Steel Creek Valley, Roark Bluff upriver to the west, and a half-mile bluff extending downstream to the north.

One of the best short hikes in the Buffalo National River is a few miles west of Steel Creek at Lost Valley. There you can hike the 2-mile Lost Valley Trail to Eden Falls, a cascade tumbling 170 feet at the head of the canyon. Admire it a bit from below and then take the trail up to near its top, where you'll find Eden Cave. Much of the flow for Eden Falls gurgles out of this opening in the bluff. Bring a flashlight—if you crawl into the cave, you're in for a treat. The cave quickly narrows down to a wide, low crawl space, where a short scramble on all fours leads to a 30-foot-tall chamber with a waterfall pouring from the ceiling. Along the way to Eden Falls you'll pass the Jig Saw Blocks, huge chunks of stone with contours matching the wall from which they fell; Cob Cave, which centuries ago sheltered American Indians; and a natural bridge.

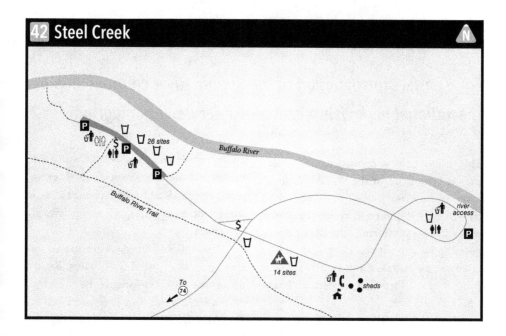

42 Steel Creek

26 sites

Buffalo River

Buffalo River Trail

river access

14 sites

sheds

To 74

Another spectacular sight near Steel Creek is Whitaker Point, better known as Hawksbill Crag, in the Upper Buffalo Wilderness. Photos of the crag have been on the cover of *National Geographic,* in outdoor product advertisements, and in lots of Arkansas Tourism literature. To get there from Ponca, take AR 43 west to AR 21, and then go south 2 miles to the Buffalo River Bridge. Turn right on Cave Mountain Road, an unmarked gravel road just before the bridge. It climbs steeply up onto Cave Mountain and follows a ridge 6 miles to a trailhead on the right. It's a 1.5-mile hike to Hawksbill Crag, a huge cliff with a rock overhang above the Upper Buffalo Wilderness. You can walk right out onto the crag and be awed by the view over the upper reaches of the Buffalo River spread out below.

:: Getting There

From Ponca drive 1 mile east on AR 74. At the top of the long climb from Ponca, the entrance to Steel Creek will be on your left. Take this winding and steep paved road 1 mile to Steel Creek. The equestrian camp will be immediately to your right. To reach the main camp, take the left fork at the bottom of the hill and drive 0.5 mile to the campground.

GPS COORDINATES   N 36° 1.809'   W 93° 20.509'

43

Tyler Bend

For a perfect introduction to the Buffalo River country, stop by the national park visitor center at Tyler Bend Campground.

This picturesque campground is nestled in Tyler Bend of the Buffalo National River. If the Army Corps of Engineers had had its way, Tyler Bend would be under water. Just downstream is the site of a proposed 1960s dam site on the Buffalo. Plans to drown the Buffalo River country sparked conservation efforts that created this beautiful national park.

Tyler Bend's visitor center is a wonderful introduction to the Buffalo River country. In addition to books, maps, and various exhibits, the center shows a movie covering the geology, wildlife, and history of the area. The film includes interviews with descendants of original settlers in the rugged country along the Buffalo. Their stories bring to life the haunting tumbledown homesteads scattered throughout the park.

The campground is in an open area that was once farm fields. Consequently, it does not yet have good shade in all sites, but the National Park Service has planted many trees that provide better cover with each passing season. The trees grown quite a bit since the previous edition of this book in

2005, providing much more shady space than before. All sites are spacious, level, grassy, and nicely landscaped, with picnic tables on stone pads. Sites 9, 12, 13, 19, and 22 have the best shade.

The walk-in campsites are spaced farther apart than the drive-in sites. Backed up against the trees fringing the river, they offer a little shade and have more privacy than the drive-in sites. A grassy expanse between the walk-ins and their parking area is a perfect place for sunbathing or tossing a Frisbee. I like the walk-in sites best, especially site J at the far south end of the campground, as well as A and D to the north.

Though the campground here is a bit overdeveloped, I included it because there is much to do in the area. For starters, canoeing above and below Tyler Bend is wonderful. Downstream from camp the Buffalo is usually floatable year-round. From Tyler Bend to the river village of Gilbert is an easy 5.6-mile float. On the way you'll drift around horseshoe-shaped Lane Bend, a 2.5-mile meander that you could cross on a quarter-mile hike. Gilbert itself is a quaint little town at the end of the road, with a general store stocked with items from today as well as antiques.

For a longer float, shuttle upstream to Woolum Ford and paddle the 15 miles back to Tyler Bend. In spring, when the river flows faster, you can make this trip in a day, coasting beneath majestic bluffs that tower

:: Ratings

BEAUTY: ★ ★ ★ ★ ★
PRIVACY: ★ ★ ★
SPACIOUSNESS: ★ ★ ★ ★ ★
QUIET: ★ ★ ★ ★
SECURITY: ★ ★ ★ ★ ★
CLEANLINESS: ★ ★ ★ ★ ★

:: Key Information

ADDRESS: Route 1, Box 46, St. Joe, AR 72675

OPERATED BY: National Park Service

CONTACT: 870-439-2502; nps.gov/buff

OPEN: Year-round

SITES: 28 drive-in, 10 walk-in, 5 group

SITE AMENITIES: Table, fire pit with grate, lantern pole

ASSIGNMENT: First come, first served; reservations required for group sites

REGISTRATION: Self-pay at campground entrance

FACILITIES: Mid-Mar.-mid-Nov.: Water, flush toilets, showers, dump station; Year-round: Amphitheater, pavilion, picnic area, visitor center, phone

PARKING: At drive-in sites; adjacent lots for group and walk-in sites

FEE: $12 individual, $3 per person for group with $33 minimum

ELEVATION: 600'

RESTRICTIONS:

■ **Pets:** On 6-foot leash at campground; not allowed on trails

■ **Fires:** In fire pits; burn only wood gathered or purchased locally

■ **Alcohol:** Allowed, subject to Arkansas state laws

■ **Vehicles:** Up to 40 feet

■ **Other:** 14-day stay limit; 6-person limit per site; no glass containers in river, in caves, within 100 feet of streams, or on trails

over eight bends in the serpentine course of the Buffalo.

Six miles of trails await you at Tyler Bend. You can add miles by hiking the Buffalo River Trail east and west of the Tyler Bend trail system. Going west, the Buffalo River Trail connects to the Ozark Highlands Trail at Woolum Ford, where you can hike almost 200 miles west to Lake Fort Smith. Trailheads are next to the amphitheater, next to the visitor center, and at the Collier Homestead a mile up the entrance road.

The prettiest hike at Tyler Bend is the River View Trail, a half-mile stretch on bluffs above the river upstream from the campground. Depending upon which trailhead and connecting trails you choose, you can hike this path above the river on loops ranging in length from 1 to 4 miles. Besides passing spectacular views, the River View Trail loops also visit the nearly intact house at the Collier Homestead. Flowers still

bloom in the yard so many springs after the Colliers left. When you see irises and daffodils blooming near an Ozarks trail, you're often near someone's abandoned homesite.

You can drive to the Collier Homestead too. The turnoff for this historic site is on the campground entrance road, and the homestead is a 100-yard walk from the parking area. From the homestead it's a half-mile hike over fairly level terrain to a breathtaking overlook of the confluence of the Buffalo River and Calf Creek. The Buffalo River Trail heads west from the Collier Trailhead too. Maps available at the visitor center or printed from the park website will guide you around Tyler Bend's trails.

If you want to do a little back-road adventuring from your campsite at Tyler Bend, find your way to Peter Cave Bluff. There you'll have a panoramic view of a hairpin bend in the Buffalo River—one of the more spectacular vistas in the park. At the point

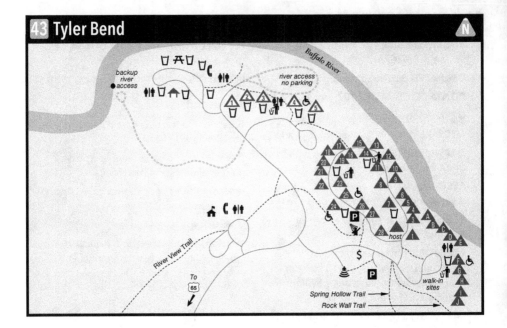

43 Tyler Bend

of the hairpin curve, there's a curiously bald spot on the bluff top. This is the Tie Slide, where railroad ties cut in the surrounding forest were once slid into the river below, and then floated downstream to Gilbert.

To get to Peter Cave Bluff, turn west onto the gravel road just south of the Collier Homestead parking area. This is Calf Creek Road, and 3.5 miles later it will take you to Peter Cave Bluff. It's a rough road with several forks and a splashing ford of Calf Creek, and it's a great mountain bike ride. It can be a little hairy in a car, but I've made it several times in my Mazda 626, so you can too. Just don't ford Calf Creek in your car if it's too deep. Bring the Trails Illustrated *Buffalo River East Half* map (available at the visitor center) to help you choose the correct turns at each fork. Once at the magnificent bluff, you'll be glad you made the effort to get there.

:: Getting There

Head 30 miles southeast of Harrison on US 65. The Tyler Bend entrance is at Silver Hill, marked by a big brown sign. Turn west off US 65 and follow the paved road 3 miles to the campground.

GPS COORDINATES N 35° 59.148' W 92° 45.764'

Ozark National Forest

44

Blanchard Springs Recreation Area

Blanchard Springs Recreation Area's caverns, springs, swimming holes, and towering pines cool you on the hottest summer day.

Blanchard Springs Recreation Area, hidden away deep in a narrow forested valley, is one of the most beautiful campgrounds in the Ozark Mountains. Though Blanchard Springs is a popular destination, the campground is at the far end of the complex, where it's peaceful even on the busiest weekend. Sylamore Creek, a clear spring-fed stream, meanders through camp, paralleled by the Sylamore Creek Trail. There are two swimming holes in the creek, miles of trails to hike and mountain bike, and caverns to explore. The nearby Ozark Folk Center is a wonderful place to learn about Ozark Mountain history and traditions.

As you enter Blanchard Springs, you'll get a quick tour of the area, passing the caverns on the descent from AR 14. Turn left at the T at the bottom of the hill, drive past the picnic area and swimming hole, and cross Sylamore Creek into the campground's lower loop. Closed indefinitely after floods

pounded many Arkansas campgrounds in 2011, this loop was still shut down as this book went to press. After U.S. Forest Service evaluation, it may be opened in the future. If so, here's what you'll find there. Sites 1–8, which are packed a little too close together, are on a spur to the right of the campground entrance. To the left are sites 9–13, with much better spacing between each camp. Sites 9, 11, and 14 are choice sites next to Sylamore Creek.

To reach the best campsites, drive past site 14, splash through the creek on a concrete slab, and pull into the lower campground loop with sites 16–31. This remote loop at the far end of the complex is very quiet, has secluded sites, and even has its own swimming hole near the loop entrance. Sites 16, 19, 20, and 21 are wonderful camping spots on the banks of Sylamore Creek. Behind site 28 a spur trail leads to the Sylamore Creek Trail. Sites 26a and 26b form a double site for small groups and families. This back loop is definitely the place to be. Because you must ford Sylamore Creek to reach these sites, the campground is sometimes closed when heavy rains are forecast so that you won't be trapped there. A quick check of the Ozark National Forest's website before you head to Blanchard is recommended. Closures are noted on the right

:: Ratings

BEAUTY: ★ ★ ★ ★ ★
PRIVACY: ★ ★ ★ ★ ★
SPACIOUSNESS: ★ ★ ★ ★
QUIET: ★ ★ ★ ★
SECURITY: ★ ★ ★ ★
CLEANLINESS: ★ ★ ★ ★ ★

:: Key Information

ADDRESS: P.O. Box 1279, 609 Sylamore Ave., Mountain View, AR 72560

OPERATED BY: Ozark NF/Sylamore Ranger District

CONTACT: 870-269-3228 or 870-757-2211; www.fs.usda.gov/osfnf

OPEN: Year-round

SITES: 32 individual, 2 group

SITE AMENITIES: Table, fire pit with grate, lantern pole, grill

ASSIGNMENT: First come, first served

REGISTRATION: Self-pay at loop entrance

FACILITIES: Water, showers, flush toilets, bathhouse, beach, picnic area, amphitheater, pavilions, visitor center, cave tours, trails

PARKING: At each site

FEE: $10 single, $35–$60 group sites, $3 day-use fee per vehicle

ELEVATION: 400'

RESTRICTIONS:

■ **Pets:** On leash only; not allowed on beach

■ **Fires:** In fire pits; burn only wood gathered or purchased locally

■ **Alcohol:** At site only, subject to Arkansas state laws

■ **Vehicles:** Up to 32 feet

■ **Other:** 5-night stay limit in summer, 14-night stay limit rest of year; 6-person limit per site; no glass containers on beach or in creek; no jumping off rocks

side of the home page under the heading "Alerts and Warnings."

Blanchard Springs is the perfect antidote to the heat and humidity of an Arkansas summer. Stately old pines and hardwoods shade all sites. Just downstream from the campground is a great swimming hole, complete with a gravel beach, bathhouse, picnic sites, and impressive rock outcrops. After your swim, go to the picnic area and check out Shelter Cave, a deep undercut hideout at the base of a tall bluff.

Another place to beat the heat is Blanchard Springs, at the opposite end of the recreation area from the campground. A paved trail with beautiful stonework bridges, walls, and steps leads out to a low bluff in the hillside where the spring tumbles from its outlet and splashes into a pool. Gushing 5,000 chilly gallons per minute, the spring water cools the hollow below the outlet before it's caught in Mirror Lake just downstream. The cold waters of

the lake are home to a trout population just waiting for you to try your luck.

The coolest place in the park is Blanchard Springs Caverns, a living cave where formations are still growing. The caverns showcase otherworldly stalactites, stalagmites, columns, walls of flowstone, and underground lakes and streams that feed the spring you just visited. The visitor center offers exhibits and a movie about the cave's development and geologic history, and guided tours are available to lead you through the caverns' wonders. The Dripstone Trail Tour is an easy half-mile tour through a series of grand rooms full of cave formations. The Discovery Trail Tour goes deeper into the caverns. Covering 1.2 miles and more than 200 stairsteps, this strenuous tour is well worth the effort. On the Discovery Trail you'll see underground lakes in the caverns' third level, check out the cave's natural entrance, and see fantastic crystalline formations. The Wild Cave Tour is for real adventurers. It requires crawling, climbing, and slithering under low ceilings. You'll be a true spelunker, exploring Blanchard Springs Caverns in hard hats and kneepads and carrying your own lights.

If you prefer the outdoors to the underground, Blanchard Springs is a great place for hiking and biking. Mountain bikers will love the Syllamo Mountain Bike Trail, a five-loop, 50-mile singletrack network north and east of Blanchard Springs. The Syllamo's 4.3-mile White River Bluff Loop has some difficult sections, but it is the most scenic ride on the network. The tougher 7.3-mile Bald Scrappy Loop is fine for beginners who don't mind walking their bikes through some challenging sections. The 12-mile Scrappy Mountain Loop, recommended for advanced riders only, is the hardest trail. Beginners should ride the Bad Branch Loop, 12 miles of relatively easy singletrack. The 14-mile Jack's Branch Loop can be accessed right from camp, but much of its southern half requires advanced mountain biking skills. Maps of

the Syllamo are available at the caverns visitor center and on the forest's website.

If biking's not for you, take a hike on the 24-mile Sylamore Creek Trail. It begins near the White River 5 miles east of camp and runs through Blanchard Springs to Barkshed Recreation Area 9 miles to the west, following the clear pools and riffles of North Sylamore Creek the entire way. A good destination is Gunner Pool Recreation Area, 5 trail miles west of Blanchard Springs. Site of the Civilian Conservation Corps Camp Hedges in the 1930s, Gunner Pool, with cliffs overlooking North Sylamore Creek, must have been a great place to live and work. The last mile before Gunner Pool has impressive bluffs and vistas. The Sylamore Creek Trail to Barkshed continues past more bluffs, creeks, and hollows just as pretty as those you'll see on your way to Gunner Pool. From Barkshed, the trail continues an additional 10 miles northwest and connects with the Sylamore section of the Ozark Highlands Trail at the Cripple Turkey Trailhead.

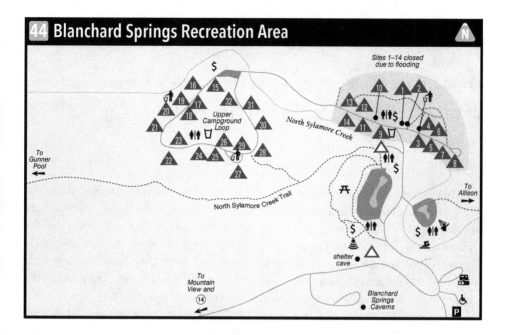

:: Getting There

Drive 12 miles northwest of Mountain View on AR 14. The entrance to Blanchard Springs will be on the right. The visitor center and caverns are 1.5 miles down the road, and the campground and recreation area are another 1.5 miles past the visitor center.

GPS COORDINATES   N 35° 57.592'   W 92° 12.053'

45

Gunner Pool Recreation Area

From Gunner Pool you can hike the North Sylamore Trail or enjoy wading and splashing in the cool waters of Sylamore Creek.

The pleasant campground at Gunner Pool Recreation Area isn't just another excellent facility built during the Great Depression by the Civilian Conservation Corps—it's the old site of an actual CCC camp. More than 2,200 young men went through what was then known as Camp Hedges, home of Company 743. A normal complement of 170 enrollees worked here at this streamside hideaway in the Ozarks.

Little remains of the old CCC camp, but when you settle in at Gunner Pool, you'll wish that you could spend as much time here as the CCC did (without the work, of course). North Sylamore Creek trickles through camp, overlooked by low bluffs next to the lower campground. Gunner Pool, namesake for this comfortable spot, is a small lake on a side stream of North Sylamore Creek. Though Forest Service Road 2011/Gunner Pool Road passes through the campground, there is little traffic to disrupt the calm at Gunner Pool. A fine grove of trees makes nearly every campsite a shady one.

:: Ratings

BEAUTY: ★ ★ ★ ★ ★
PRIVACY: ★ ★ ★ ★
SPACIOUSNESS: ★ ★ ★
QUIET: ★ ★ ★ ★
SECURITY: ★ ★ ★ ★
CLEANLINESS: ★ ★ ★ ★ ★

Gunner Pool's campsites are divided into three areas. Sites 1–14 are on either side of a loop east of FS 1102 as you enter the recreation area. Most sites are adequately separated from their neighbors by good spacing and belts of trees. Sites 2 and 3 offer the best privacy on this loop. Sites 4 and 5 and sites 6 and 7 are paired campsites on spurs 100 feet off the main loop, with tent and table pads terraced into the hillside. While these paired sites are very close to each other, they are secluded from the others on the loop. They are perfect for small groups wishing to camp together. Sites 1, 9, 10, and 14 are spacious sites in the middle of the loop and are ideal camping spots for stargazers.

Across the road from sites 1–14 are three walk-in sites next to a small picnic area. Numbered T-1, T-2, and T-3, they're nice spots with lots of open space. Just north of the picnic sites is a second loop, containing sites 15–19. Site 16 is a nice spot next to Gunner Pool's dam. Campsites 17 and 18 are roomy and located on the outside of this small loop. On the fringe of the campground, with views of the pool, they are the most private sites in the campground.

Sites 20–24 are the most popular camping spots at Gunner Pool. Located below the main campground on a spur road next to North Sylamore Creek, they are the prettiest sites in camp. A bluff towers over the creek and these campsites. Site 21 is my

:: Key Information

ADDRESS: P.O. Box 1279, 609 Sylamore Ave., Mountain View, AR 72560

OPERATED BY: Ozark NF/Sylamore Ranger District

CONTACT: 870-269-3228 or 870-757-2211; www.fs.usda.gov/osfnf

OPEN: Year-round

SITES: 27

SITE AMENITIES: Table, fire pit with grate, lantern pole, tent pad; some with barbecue grill

ASSIGNMENT: First come, first served

REGISTRATION: Self-pay in center of upper campground

FACILITIES: Water (except in winter), vault toilets, picnic area, trails

PARKING: At each site

FEE: $7

ELEVATION: 480'

RESTRICTIONS:

■ **Pets:** On leash only

■ **Fires:** In fire pits; burn only wood gathered or purchased locally

■ **Alcohol:** At site only

■ **Vehicles:** Up to 25 feet; steep and winding road not recommended for large RVs

■ **Other:** 14-day stay limit; no glass containers in North Sylamore Creek

pick in the lower area. At the end of the road and close to the stream, it's shaded and private. Sites 22 and 23 are nice spots close to the stream, but other campers might pass through on their way to North Sylamore Creek.

Splashing in the creek is a fine way to while away the hours at Gunner Pool. So is relaxing in your campsite reading, writing, or shooting the breeze. This campground is popular in summer, often filling on weekends when school is out. It's also busy in October, when fall colors and festivals in nearby Mountain View attract travelers to the area.

I like Gunner Pool in winter or early spring, when I have it to myself. Those seasons are best for my favorite activity—hiking the Ozark trails. The 24-mile North Sylamore Creek Trail passes right through Gunner Pool. A quarter-mile walk south of camp goes to an overlook from the bluffs above the creek. Hiking 5 miles south, you'll pass several scenic spots on your way to Blanchard

Springs—an attractive day-use area and campground where you can cool down on an underground tour of Blanchard Springs Caverns (see profile on page 146).

A 4-mile hike northwest from camp goes to Barkshed Recreation Area, a wonderful place to end a hike on a hot day. North Sylamore Creek has a pretty swimming hole below a small bluff at Barkshed. If you can't hike that far, drive or bike the wooded forest roads to Barkshed and check out this great spot. There's a campground at Barkshed, but it's not as nice as Gunner Pool.

While you're at Gunner Pool, drive 15 miles east to Mountain View and wander around Ozark Folk Center State Park. It showcases the heritage of the Ozark Mountain region with crafts demonstrations, music, cooking, and more. During tourist season (mid-April–early November) you can enjoy concerts and watch artisans demonstrate crafts such as pottery, quilting, blacksmithing, and other skills needed

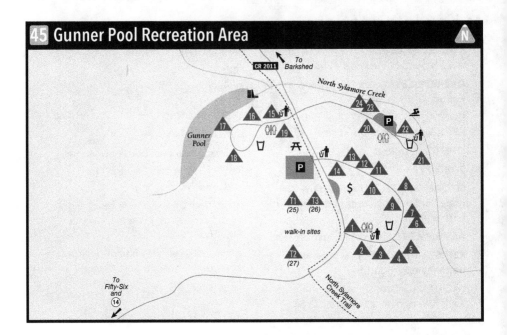

to survive the old times in the Ozarks. To really get into the Ozarks culture, take one of the workshops on dulcimer, banjo, and Autoharp. After class, come back to camp and practice by the fire until the wee hours. Quietly, of course.

:: Getting There

From the west edge of Fifty-Six, turn north on Forest Service Road 1102/Gunner Pool Road and drive 3 miles to Gunner Pool. A sign just west of town marks the turn, and the road goes right through camp.

GPS COORDINATES N 35° 59.666' W 92° 12.745'

46

Haw Creek Falls Recreation Area

This campground is next to the 15,000-acre Hurricane Creek Wilderness and its beautiful natural bridge.

The word *haw* is old-time mule-driver jargon. The driver would shout "Haw" to turn his team left, and "Gee" to turn it right. Gee Creek runs into Haw Creek near Haw Creek Falls Recreation Area, and at their junction Gee Creek flows from the right and Haw Creek from the left. From this confluence just upstream from the campground, Haw Creek flows over lovely cascades next to camp on its way to nearby Big Piney Creek.

No longer is anyone calling mule-team commands in this quiet campground on Haw Creek. A thick canopy of hardwoods shades all sites, and walls of trees separate each campsite from its neighbors. Distances between sites are just right, and several sites overlook Haw Creek. In addition to the usual table, fire grate, and lantern pole, all sites sport fire rings, barbecue grills, and attractive stone-outlined tables and tent pads. The well pump in the campground has been locked off, so there's no water in camp. However, the camping fee was reduced, which makes Haw Creek one of the best camping deals around.

:: Ratings

BEAUTY: ★ ★ ★ ★ ★
PRIVACY: ★ ★ ★ ★
SPACIOUSNESS: ★ ★ ★
QUIET: ★ ★ ★ ★ ★
SECURITY: ★ ★ ★ ★
CLEANLINESS: ★ ★ ★ ★

Sites 1–5 are all nice sites on the side of the loop away from Haw Creek. The really good ones, though, start with site 6, a very private site with scattered boulders for sitting or organizing your stuff. Site 7 is on the end of the loop with lots of space separating it from the other sites. Site 8, a pull-through on the creek side of the loop, is my favorite. It has tons of room and great shade, and it's right next to Haw Creek Falls. Stone steps lead to the falls just north of the site. Site 9, another pull-through, is just beyond site 8. It's another good spot with close proximity to the falls.

Haw Creek Falls Recreation Area is a nice place any time of year, but it's especially pretty in spring, when the creek is flowing deep. You'll know how it's running when you pull into camp and splash across it on a concrete slab. When the creek is up, the waterfall next to the campground comes alive—you'll fall asleep to the sound of its roar. The falls are wide ledges in the creek with several pour-offs and pools. Unless the creek is flooding, it's easy to pick your way out to the middle of the stream to photograph the falls, wade the creek, swim in its two deep pools, or just laze in the sun on the huge rock slabs in the streambed.

Haw Creek pours into Big Piney Creek a mile downstream from the camp. Bring your raft, whitewater canoe, or kayak to paddle the Class I–III rapids of this Wild and Scenic

:: Key Information

ADDRESS: 12000 SR 27, Hector, AR 72843

OPERATED BY: Ozark NF/Big Piney Ranger District

CONTACT: 479-284-3150; www.fs.usda.gov/osfnf

OPEN: Year-round

SITES: 9

SITE AMENITIES: Table, fire pit with grate, lantern pole, tent pad, barbecue grill, fire ring

ASSIGNMENT: First come, first served

REGISTRATION: Self-pay at loop entrance

FACILITIES: Vault toilets, trail; no drinking water available

PARKING: At each site

FEE: $4

ELEVATION: 1,000'

RESTRICTIONS:

■ **Pets:** On leash only

■ **Fires:** In fire pits; burn only wood gathered or purchased locally

■ **Alcohol:** At site only

■ **Vehicles:** Up to 22 feet

■ **Other:** 14-day stay limit; no glass containers in creek

River. It's an 8-mile trip from AR 123 to Treat, and an 18-mile run to Long Pool. Water levels are normally suitable in spring or after downpours. When the creek is too low to boat, try your luck fishing the Big Piney. Not many folks fish the creek's populations of sunfish, catfish, and several varieties of bass, so the angling is often great. When stream levels are low, you can hike along the creek bed, fishing deep pools and riffles along the Big Piney.

If you want to see some really cool stuff, get on the Ozark Highlands Trail and make tracks into the Hurricane Creek Wilderness. Covering 15,000 acres north of AR 123 on the east side of Big Piney Creek, this wilderness protects the headwaters of Hurricane Creek and hides a beautiful natural bridge. The bridge is a 6-mile trek from the Big Piney Trailhead, which is a mile east of camp, so save your energy by starting from the trailhead instead of the campground. The trailhead is at the abandoned Fort Douglas School, and you can check out this historic old building before or after your hike.

Four miles into the wilderness you'll come to a fork. Stay left—the right fork is the high-water route for hikers to avoid Hurricane Creek when it's in flood stage. It misses all the good scenery, including the bridge. A mile down the left fork you'll cross Hurricane Creek, climb to an old road, and turn right to follow it. The trail soon parallels a bluff. Keep your eye on the bluff, and a half mile after crossing Hurricane Creek you'll see the natural bridge high in the cliff.

It's worth the trip just to see the bridge, but don't turn around yet. In the next half mile the trail goes past a huge boulder and back down to Hurricane Creek. There you'll find a scenic area with backpacker campsites next to the creek and rocks to lounge on while you enjoy the view. It's a perfect spot to relax and snack before heading back to the trailhead.

If you're feeling energetic or can arrange a shuttle, hike the 13 miles across the wilderness area and follow the spur to a trailhead at the old townsite of Chancel. On the spur you'll

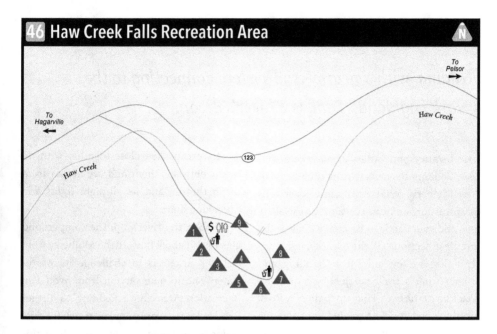

46 Haw Creek Falls Recreation Area

hike several hundred feet along an unbeliev-ably well-crafted rock wall next to a field. As hard as farming must have been back in these deep woods, some homesteader found time to build this impressive wall instead of just piling rocks at his field edge.

:: Getting There

From Pelsor on AR 7, drive west 12 miles on AR 123. Haw Creek Falls Recreation Area will be on the south side of the road.

GPS COORDINATES   N 35° 40.762'   W 93° 15.585'

47

Redding Recreation Area

Redding, with a nearby trail system connecting to the Ozark Highlands Trail, is a hiker's dream.

For beauty and variety of outdoor activities, Redding Recreation Area can't be beat. The Mulberry Wild and Scenic River rolls past this forested camp, waiting to swallow you and your canoe in its rapids. One of the prettiest sections of the Ozark Highlands Trail passes a few miles from Redding, and a spur from a trailhead just east of camp leads up to the trail. Hike up to the Spy Rock overlook and you'll be treated to panoramic views of the Mulberry River Valley. If you continue along the Ozark Highlands Trail to Hare Mountain, you'll be on the highest point along the whole trail, with vistas to match the altitude.

Redding Recreation Area is a nice place to be. All sites are well shaded and spacious. Most are separated from neighboring camps by thick woods and brush. They're spaced far enough apart to ensure privacy but close enough for you to socialize with your neighbors if you want. Water spigots are scattered throughout the campground, and it's only a short walk to hot showers and flush toilets. The only sites to avoid are 19, 20, and 21—they're packed close together with no brush between them and are across from the bathroom and its all-night lights and squeaking door.

When the river's up, the campground gets busy. People flock to the Mulberry from all over Arkansas to challenge its whitewater. The 16-mile section from Wolf Pen Recreation Area above Redding to Turner Bend below is a very popular stretch for river runners. Dropping 13–15 feet per mile on this run, the Mulberry roars through sharp turns, cascades over rock ledges, pushes through strainers and willow thickets, and smashes over boulders. It's a blast to paddle—with sets of rapids named Jump Start, Whoop and Holler, and Big Al's Twist, how could it ever be boring?

Gradients ease below Turner Bend, but the Mulberry is still a challenge when it's up. It's a 10.6-mile run from Turner Bend to Campbell Cemetery, and 12.7 miles from Campbell Cemetery to Mill Creek. Water levels are usually suitable from late fall to early June. Shuttles and canoe rentals are available nearby at Turner Bend Country Store or at Byrd's Adventure Center. Turner Bend Store has something that might make your campout a bit more cultured—a nice selection of local wines and ice-cold beer.

If you don't mind dust and rough roads, take a drive on U.S. Forest Service roads in the surrounding Ozark National Forest. From Cass it's a 17-mile drive on White Rock

:: Ratings

BEAUTY: ★ ★ ★ ★
PRIVACY: ★ ★ ★ ★ ★
SPACIOUSNESS: ★ ★ ★ ★ ★
QUIET: ★ ★ ★ ★
SECURITY: ★ ★ ★ ★
CLEANLINESS: ★ ★ ★ ★ ★

:: Key Information

ADDRESS: 2591 AR 21, Clarksville, AR 72830

OPERATED BY: Ozark NF/Pleasant Hill Ranger District

CONTACT: 479-754-2864; www.fs.usda.gov/osfnf

OPEN: Year-round

SITES: 24

SITE AMENITIES: Table, fire pit with grate, lantern pole, tent pad

ASSIGNMENT: First come, first served

REGISTRATION: Self-pay at loop entrance

FACILITIES: Water, flush toilets, showers, river access, trails

PARKING: At each site; $3 per vehicle day-use fee

FEE: $10

ELEVATION: 760'

RESTRICTIONS:

- **Pets:** On leash only
- **Fires:** In fire pits; burn only wood gathered or purchased locally
- **Alcohol:** At site only
- **Vehicles:** Up to 35 feet
- **Other:** 14-day stay limit; no glass containers in river

Mountain Road/Forest Service Road 1003 to White Rock Mountain, one of the more scenic spots in the Boston Mountains. Along the way you'll pass Gray's Spring, a mountainside picnic area, and squeeze through Bee Rock, a massive split boulder. Because it's always a few degrees cooler there, the summit of White Rock Mountain is a nice summer destination (see profile on page 165 for more information). A 2-mile hike circumnavigates the edge of this flat-topped peak, and from an overlook in the picnic area there's a 270-degree panoramic vista of the surrounding mountains. After admiring the view, coast down the mountainside to Shores Lake, a Civilian Conservation Corps lake with good fishing and a nice swimming beach. From Shores Lake it's 10 miles back to Cass on Baptist Village Road, completing a 40-mile drive in a rugged mountain landscape.

For a technical mountain biking challenge, take your bike over to the Mill Creek ATV area south of Combs. This 42-mile trail system features a 27-mile main loop interlaced with 15 miles of interior loops and connectors. It varies from laid-back cruises on ridges and stream bottoms to thigh-burning climbs and white-knuckle descents. Except for the easy Burrel Mountain Loop, Mill Creek is only for strong and experienced riders.

If road riding is more your thing, there's wonderful biking right from camp at Redding. AR 215 is a quiet laid-back highway paralleling the Mulberry River, and a 16-mile ride east from camp takes you to the Oark General Store and Café. Established in 1890, it's the oldest continually operating store in Arkansas. Though it does carry minimal groceries, it's more of a café than a store these days, and it serves wonderful burgers, pies, and hand-dipped ice cream cones. If the 32-mile round-trip between Redding and Oark isn't quite enough for you, continue east another 5 miles to Catalpa. The pavement ends there, and another café awaits.

For hikers, Redding is a dream. The Redding–Spy Rock Loop leaves from a trailhead a half mile east of the campground. This 9-mile loop climbs the side of Morgan

47 Redding Recreation Area

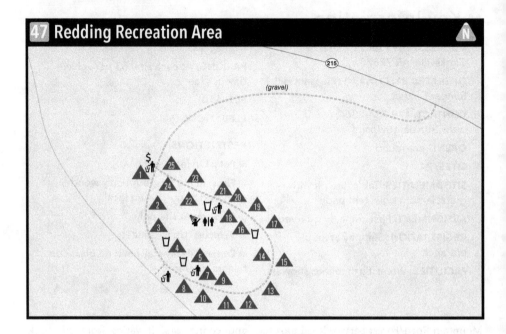

Mountain to Spy Rock Vista and returns, passing several small waterfalls along the way. Near Spy Rock a connector runs over to the Ozark Highlands Trail, tying you into nearly 200 miles of scenic wandering.

The 19-mile section of the Ozark Highlands Trail between Cherry Bend on AR 23 and Lick Branch Trailhead on County Road 33 is gorgeous. It goes right over 2,380-foot Hare Mountain, the highest point on this 180-mile trail. An old well and a haunting rock wall are all that remain of a farm that once worked this flat-topped mountain. The old wall is an ideal seat for admiring the valley of the Mulberry and surrounding Boston Mountains fading into the distant smoky blue haze. The rest of this section of trail travels bluff edges, splashes through streams, skirts waterfalls on Indian Creek, and passes through the Marinoni Scenic Area, a fantastic little canyon not far from Lick Branch.

For an easy hike to the peak of Hare Mountain, use the Hare Mountain Trailhead 4 miles up Morgan Mountain Road from AR 215. From there it's only a 2-mile hike on a razorback ridge to the top of Hare Mountain.

:: Getting There

From Ozark drive 18 miles north on AR 23 to AR 215. Drive 3 miles east on AR 215 to the campground on the south side of the highway.

GPS COORDINATES N 35° 40.794' W 93° 46.635'

48

Richland Creek Recreation Area

Hike from your campsite to Twin Falls, possibly the most beautiful waterfall in the Ozarks.

Located 9 miles from the nearest paved road, Richland Creek is a little backwoods campground that packs quite an outdoor punch. There are trails to hike, a wonderful swimming hole, wilderness waterfalls to explore, and winding, hilly forest roads to mountain bike. Even the drive into the campground is wonderful—Forest Service Road 1205 is called Falling Water Road, and you'll know why if you make the drive when the creeks are flowing. Best of all, the rugged road to camp keeps RVs from getting to Richland Creek.

Richland Creek used to be a charming and kind of disorganized little place—a bit scruffy, but a wonderful free campground way back in the mountains. As this edition went to press in late 2013, however, Richland was being completely refurbished. Since the rebuild wasn't complete at that time, there may be a few inaccuracies in this somewhat vague description. The forest service had yet to set a fee for camping at Richland Creek's upgraded sites, but this campground deep in the Ozark woods is still a wonderful place to escape from the outside world, even if it is all spruced up and now charges for camping.

All sites in the campground are now on the bench above Richland Creek. The old streamside campsites have been converted to day-use areas accessible only by foot, either by walking down the gated road near the pumphouse or via stairs from the camp. There are 16 single sites and one double site scattered along both sides of a tadpole-shaped loop that starts near the pumphouse. Sites are well spaced from each other on 30- to 40-foot spurs, and most are well shaded. Site 9 on the inside of the loop and sites 15–17 at its end offer the least shade, but they'd make great camping spots in fall and winter when a little sunshine is welcome. Sites along the loop's north side are closest to Richland Creek and its swimming hole, and sites 8, 9, and 10 at the back of the loop are near Falling Water Creek.

Though it's way off the beaten path, this popular campground often fills on weekends from spring through fall, and on holiday weekends it's jammed. Plan accordingly and visit Richland Creek during the week or in off-season. Most folks come to hike deep into the Richland Creek Wilderness immediately west of camp and check out Twin Falls. There's a day-use parking area just east

:: Ratings

BEAUTY: ★ ★ ★ ★ ★
PRIVACY: ★ ★ ★ ★
SPACIOUSNESS: ★ ★ ★ ★
QUIET: ★ ★ ★ ★ ★
SECURITY: ★ ★ ★ ★
CLEANLINESS: ★ ★ ★ ★

:: Key Information

ADDRESS: AR 7 N., Jasper, AR 72641

OPERATED BY: Ozark NF/Big Piney Ranger District

CONTACT: 870-446-5122; www.fs.usda.gov/osfnf

OPEN: Year-round

SITES: 16 single, 1 double

SITE AMENITIES: Table, lantern pole, fire pit with grate

ASSIGNMENT: First come, first served

REGISTRATION: At pay station near entrance

FACILITIES: Vault toilets, trails, swimming hole; water (Apr.-Nov. only)

PARKING: At each site

FEE: Not available at press time but will likely range from $7-10 single, $15-18 double, $3-5 day-use fee

ELEVATION: 1,000'

RESTRICTIONS:

■ **Pets:** On leash only

■ **Fires:** In fire pits and fire rings; burn only wood gathered or purchased locally

■ **Alcohol:** At site only

■ **Vehicles:** Up to 30 feet

■ **Other:** 14-day stay limit; no glass containers in creek

of the camp loop for hikers heading into the wilderness and folks coming to swim in the creek or picnic on its banks.

There's no official trail to the wilderness area's waterfalls—just a mishmash of paths following Richland Creek into the wilderness. Simply go to the end of the day-use area, cross Falling Water Creek, and start working your way upstream along the south side of Richland Creek. It's about 3 challenging miles to the falls, but it's so pretty that you'll love the trek. When Richland Creek takes a hard turn from the south, with another creek pouring in from the far side, you're in for some fantastic scenery. If you continue upstream on Richland Creek another half mile, you'll find a waterfall where the creek pours over a 100-foot-wide ledge.

Devil's Fork, that other stream pouring into Richland Creek, has the even more spectacular Twin Falls. A quarter mile upstream from Devil's Fork's junction with Richland Creek, Big Devil's Fork and Long Devil's Fork come together as a stunning

pair of waterfalls, pouring into a broad pool from opposite sides of a low bluff. These falls are broad, 15-foot-tall curtains pouring off deeply undercut ledges.

More hiking awaits you on the Ozark Highlands Trail. It comes to Richland from the south and heads east. I like the 8-mile stretch of trail from Richland Creek to the Stack Rock Trailhead on FS 1201. You'll not see anything as spectacular as Twin Falls, but it's a hike with vistas of the Richland Creek Valley, house-size boulders, rugged rock gardens, and exquisite little streams with pools and small waterfalls. If you're really energetic or can have someone shuttle you, hike the Ozark Highlands Trail clear to Woolum Ford on the Buffalo National River.

The most fun way to get to Woolum Ford is by mountain bike. It's 19 miles via FS 1205, FS 1201, and the county road heading north from the old townsite of Eula. You'll have a stiff climb and an exhilarating descent each way, two fords of Richland Creek, and lots of scenery. As you approach the Buffalo in the Richland Creek Valley, a rock wall rises on

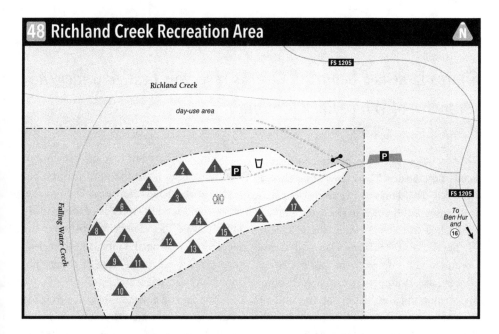

48 Richland Creek Recreation Area

your left. Ditch your bike and find your way up the rock wall and you'll be standing on The Nars, a causeway-like spine of stone with the Buffalo rolling by on the other side. At places The Nars are only a few feet wide. You can drive to Woolum and The Nars, but be careful—the stream crossings are a bit deep for some vehicles when Richland Creek is flowing strongly.

Another nearby scenic spot is Sam's Throne, a bluff-lined mountaintop that has become a rock climber's mecca. To reach Sam's Throne, drive south from Mt. Judea on AR 123. After an incredibly crooked, hilly, and beautiful 4-mile drive, the entrance to Sam's Throne will be on your right. There's parking here, but follow the gravel road several hundred yards to a second parking area. Short trails fan out from this lot to the surrounding cliff faces. You don't need to be a climber to enjoy Sam's Throne—hikers wandering out to its steep cliffs will be rewarded with sweeping views of the surrounding Ozark hills and valleys.

:: Getting There

From Pelsor at the junction of AR 7, AR 123, and AR 16, drive 8 miles east on AR 16 to Forest Service Road 1205/County Road 68, 1 mile past Ben Hur. Turn left on FS 1205/CR 68 and follow it 8.5 miles to Richland Creek Recreation Area on the left side of the road. It's easy to miss the turn onto FS 1205. If you do, go 2 miles farther on AR 16 and turn left onto FS 1313/CR 18. It goes past the Falling Water Church and joins FS 1205 to the campground.

GPS COORDINATES   N 35° 47.783'   W 92° 55.822'

49

Shores Lake Recreation Area

Shores Lake is a beautiful Ozarks reservoir nestled under the ramparts of White Rock Mountain.

Shores Lake is 82 acres of sky-blue beauty deep in the Boston Mountains of northwest Arkansas. The dam was begun by the Civilian Conservation Corps in the 1930s, but left unfinished until 1958, when the U.S. Forest Service and Arkansas Fish and Game Commission completed the project. Now Shores Lake is a popular camping, fishing, and swimming destination at the end of the pavement in the Ozark National Forest. You might not want to camp here if you're superstitious—an old cemetery lies near the campground entrance—but less timid campers will love spending a few nights in this wooded lakeside retreat.

The campground is located at the upper end of Shores Lake. It's a pretty set of campsites in a double loop under a canopy of pines and hardwoods. The tent pads at each site are outlined with native stone or wooden timbers, and almost every site is level and shaded. While many trees shade the campground, there is little ground-level brush between the sites to create privacy, and spacing between sites is a bit tight. Site

12, off by itself on a low rise above the rest of the campground, has the most privacy, but it's the least shaded campsite at Shores Lake. Sites 10 and 11 on the outside of the loop are fairly private too. Campsites 16–20 on the recreation area's north loop, while a bit close together, are off to the edge of things and thus a bit more peaceful.

The lake is a wonderful place to while away a warm summer afternoon. A grassy field sloping from the bathhouse to the water's edge is a fine place to play Frisbee or nap on your blanket in the sun. A dip in the lake is only a few steps away. In the woods behind the bathhouse 28 beautiful picnic sites are situated on a spur road running along a little highland between the day-use area and the campground.

Bring your fishing tackle—Shores Lake is stocked with bass, catfish, and bluegill. Two fishing piers near the swimming area have underwater structures to attract fish. The biggest fish stay near the middle of the lake, so you'll have more success if you bring a canoe or boat (10-horsepower motor limit). Whether you fish or paddle around, you'll have fun exploring the lake by boat.

If you like adventurous canoeing, plan to float the lower portions of the nearby Mulberry River. From Turner Bend on AR 23 west of Shores Lake, it's a 10-mile run to Campbell Cemetery on Forest Service Road 1501/Shores Lake Road. Another exciting trip is the 13-mile float from Campbell Cemetery to

:: Ratings

BEAUTY: ★ ★ ★ ★
PRIVACY: ★ ★
SPACIOUSNESS: ★ ★ ★
QUIET: ★ ★ ★ ★
SECURITY: ★ ★ ★ ★
CLEANLINESS: ★ ★ ★ ★ ★

:: Key Information

ADDRESS: 18660 Bliss Ridge Rd., Mountainburg, AR 72946

OPERATED BY: Ozark NF/Boston Mountain Ranger District

CONTACT: 479-667-2191; www.fs.usda.gov/osfnf

OPEN: Year-round

SITES: 9 basic, 12 electric

SITE AMENITIES: Table, fire pit with grate, lantern pole, tent pad

ASSIGNMENT: First come, first served

REGISTRATION: At pay station at campground entrance

FACILITIES: Water, vault toilets, trail, overlook shelter, picnic area, showers, swimming beach, pavilion, boat ramp

PARKING: At each site; $3 day-use fee per vehicle for noncampers

FEE: Apr.-Nov.: $8 single, $12 single electric, $18 double electric; Dec.-Mar.: $6 single, $10 single electric, $14 double electric; $35 pavilion

ELEVATION: 675'

RESTRICTIONS:

- **Pets:** On leash only
- **Fires:** In fire pits; burn only wood gathered or purchased locally
- **Alcohol:** At site only
- **Vehicles:** Up to 40 feet

the Mill Creek access south of Shores Lake. The Wild and Scenic Mulberry will challenge you with Class II whitewater, willow thickets, and strainers as it tumbles through the Boston Mountains. The Mulberry is normally floatable from late fall to June. Canoe rentals and shuttles are available at Turner Bend (**turnerbend.com**).

If you'd rather hike than paddle, you're in luck. A trailhead for the Shores Lake–White Rock Mountain Loop is at the north edge of the campground. On this 13.5-mile hike you'll climb to the peak of White Rock Mountain, gaining 1,600 feet of altitude on the way to its 2,260-foot summit. If the weather has been wet, you'll cross numerous streams and pass several waterfalls on your way to and from the peak. On its way to White Rock the loop uses part of the Ozark Highlands Trail. On the mountaintop you'll relax in the cool highland breezes and admire the surrounding countryside before starting the easy descent back to Shores Lake. You could even make this trek a cushy overnight jaunt by renting one of the CCC-era cabins on the peak and admiring the sunset from your comfortable accommodations on top of White Rock Mountain.

If you don't mind gravel, the forest roads north and east of Shores Lake are wonderful routes for exploring the Boston Mountains on driving tours or mountain bike rides. Going 13 miles east from Shores Lake on Shores Lake Road (FS 1501) takes you to Turner Bend, where you can enjoy a cold drink at the store there. This gravel road passes an overlook above Shores Lake. From Turner Bend you can return through the highlands on White Rock Mountain Road (FS 1003), driving through Bee Rock and past Gray's Spring Picnic Area, and descending to Shores Lake Road on Mineral Hill Road (FS 1510) or Bliss Ridge Road (FS 1505). As long as you're up in the highlands, take the 3-mile side trip to White Rock Mountain and admire the view from its breezy summit. The map of the Ozark National Forest, available at the forest office in Ozark or at the Turner Bend Country Store, is an excellent guide to these roadways.

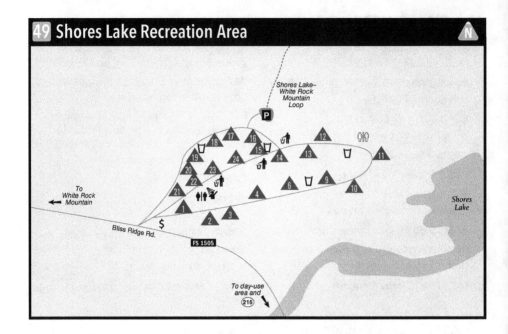

49 Shores Lake Recreation Area

Though Shores Lake is a remote hideaway in the Boston Mountains, it's a popular destination on summer weekends. If it's too busy, head for the hills on White Rock Mountain (see the following profile). The campground there is rarely full, and it's usually cooler on the mountaintop, 1,600 feet above Shores Lake.

:: Getting There

From Mulberry drive north 15 miles on AR 215 to Forest Service Road 1505/ Bliss Ridge Road. Turn left on Bliss Ridge Road and go north 0.5 mile to Shores Lake. The campground is 0.2 mile beyond the entrance to the day-use area.

GPS COORDINATES N 35° 38.608' W 93° 57.734'

50

White Rock Mountain Recreation Area

White Rock Mountain's lofty peak is a wonderful place to admire Ozark sunsets.

You don't often get to camp on top of a mountain without hiking there. Even more seldom do you enjoy incredible mountaintop vistas just a short walk from your campsite. Both of these pleasures are yours at White Rock Mountain, though you'll have to drive 10 miles of gravel roads to get there. You can see for miles during the day and enjoy cooling high-country breezes at night. It's 1,600 feet higher than the surrounding lowlands, and on the top of the 2,260-foot White Rock Mountain it's always a few degrees cooler.

White Rock is historical as well as beautiful. Its lodge, cabins, and trail shelters were built by the Civilian Conservation Corps in the 1930s. Over the years these rustic structures weathered badly. In 1987 the Friends of White Rock was formed to renovate the structures, and the renovation work was completed in 1991. The old stone and wood cabins with rock fireplaces and original furniture can be rented year-round.

Though this sounds like a commercialized place, it's really not. The nearest town is

17 miles away, and dirt roads sort out those who hate dust and bumps. The campground is on the right as you drive into the area, and the picnic area is 100 yards beyond. Each site has a stone-lined tent pad and is set well away from its neighbors. While there are enough trees to provide shade for each site, the mountaintop's thin forest with little underbrush means that all your neighbors are visible. But that's OK because this small campground doesn't feel cramped even when it's full. Sites 1–4 are between the loop and the White Rock entrance road. I prefer sites 5–8. They are on the outside of the loop, away from the road. From these sites you get hints of views through the trees, and the tent pads are set a short way down the hill for a bit more privacy. For real seclusion, set up in the group camp. It's a two-table campsite north of the main campground loop. It's a bit far from toilets and water but is the best place to be if you're looking for a little mountaintop solitude.

It's nice to hang out in the campground at White Rock and listen to the mountain breezes as they sift through the treetops. If you walk over to the picnic area and down the short spur to the trail shelter built on the cliff's edge, you can enjoy a 270-degree panorama. This shelter is a wonderful place to watch the sunset. Arrows painted on top of the wall point to local towns and give their distances from the mountaintop. At sunset,

:: Ratings

BEAUTY: ★ ★ ★ ★ ★
PRIVACY: ★ ★ ★ ★
SPACIOUSNESS: ★ ★ ★ ★ ★
QUIET: ★ ★ ★ ★ ★
SECURITY: ★ ★ ★ ★
CLEANLINESS: ★ ★ ★ ★

:: Key Information

ADDRESS: P.O. Box 76, 1803 N. 18th St., Ozark, AR 72949

OPERATED BY: Ozark NF/Boston Mountain Ranger District/White Rock Mountain Concessionaire

CONTACT: 479-667-2191, www.fs.usda.gov/osfnf; 479-369-4128, whiterockmountain.com

OPEN: Year-round

SITES: 9

SITE AMENITIES: Table, fire pit with grate, lantern pole, tent pad; some with fire rings

ASSIGNMENT: First come, first served

REGISTRATION: Pay at white house just south of campground

FACILITIES: Water, vault toilets, trail, overlook shelter, picnic area

PARKING: At each site

FEE: $10, $15 for group camp

ELEVATION: 2,250'

RESTRICTIONS:

■ **Pets:** On leash only

■ **Fires:** In fire pits; burn only wood gathered or purchased locally

■ **Alcohol:** At site only

■ **Vehicles:** Up to 22 feet

■ **Other:** 14-day stay limit; overlooks and rim trail close at sunset

just before the overlook closes, you can see the lights of each town.

To check out all the views from the peak, hike the 2.1-mile White Rock Rim Loop. It's an easy, level hike all the way around the mountaintop, with vistas almost all the way. This hike's official start is at the trailhead at the end of the cabin road, but you can pick it up from the picnic area overlook too. A mile north from the trailhead is the first of four trail shelters. This overlook is a fantastic place to greet the sunrise. Looping around to the west side there is another shelter that's only a short distance from the campground loop. Just beyond this shelter a couple of paths lead up to camp. The only drawback to this incredible hike is safety—watch your children closely on this hike, or consider not taking them on the trail at all. It follows the bluff line for most of its length, and one slip could be fatal. A sign on the entrance road warns 7 HAVE FALLEN TO THEIR DEATH.

White Rock is also part of the 14-mile Shores Lake–White Rock Mountain Loop.

This tough trail gains 1,700 feet coming up from Shores Lake. It makes a great weekend hike. You can set up camp or stash your gear in a rented cabin on White Rock Mountain, and then drive back to Shores Lake. Leave your car there and enjoy the steep climb without a pack, spend a night on the mountain, and head back to Shores Lake the next day.

Shores Lake has 82 acres of beauty and is a nice place to visit from your campsite on the mountaintop. Bring your swimsuit and fishing rod—the lake has a swimming beach and is stocked with bass, catfish, and bluegill. Two fishing piers near the beach have underwater structures to attract fish. Shores Lake has nice picnic sites, and facilities near the beach include a bathhouse where you can freshen up before heading back to camp on the top of White Rock Mountain.

If you like your water a little more wild, canoe the nearby Mulberry River. From Turner Bend on AR 23 west of Shores Lake, it's a 10-mile run to Campbell Cemetery on FS 1501. Another exciting trip is the 13-mile

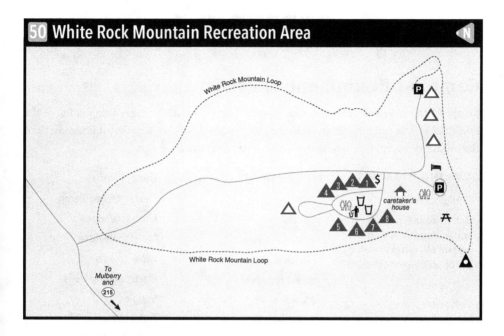

float from Campbell Cemetery to the Mill Creek access south of Shores Lake. The Wild and Scenic Mulberry will challenge you with Class II whitewater, willow thickets, and strainers as it tumbles through the Boston Mountains. The Mulberry is normally floatable from late fall to June. Canoe rentals and shuttles are available at Turner Bend.

:: Getting There

From Mulberry drive north 15 miles on AR 215 to Forest Service Road 1505/Bliss Ridge Road. Turn left on Bliss Ridge Road and go north 8 miles to FS 1003/White Rock Mountain Road. Turn left on White Rock Mountain Road and drive 1.5 miles to FS 1505/Hurricane Road. Turn right on Hurricane Road and drive 1 mile to the White Rock Mountain Recreation Area entrance. The campground is on the right as you drive into the recreation area.

GPS COORDINATES   N 35° 41.868'   W 93° 57.646'

APPENDIX A

Camping-Equipment Checklist

Except for the large and bulky items on this list, I keep a plastic storage container full of the essentials for car camping, so they're ready to go when I am. I make a last-minute check of the inventory, resupply anything that's low or missing, and away I go.

COOKING UTENSILS

Bottle opener

Bottles of salt, pepper, spices, sugar, cooking oil, and maple syrup in water-proof, spill-proof containers

Can opener

Corkscrew

Cups, plastic or tin

Dish soap (biodegradable), sponge, and towel

Fire starter

Flatware

Food of your choice

Frying pan, spatula

Fuel for stove

Lighter, matches in water-proof container

Plates

Pocketknife

Pot with lid

Stove

Tinfoil

Wooden spoon

FIRST-AID KIT

Aspirin

Band-Aids

First-aid cream

Gauze pads

Insect repellent

Moleskin

Sunscreen/lip balm

Tape, waterproof adhesive

SLEEPING GEAR

Pillow

Sleeping bag

Sleeping pad, inflatable or insulated

Tent with ground tarp and rainfly

MISCELLANEOUS

Bath soap (biodegradable), washcloth, and towel

Book(s)

Camp chair

Candles

Cooler

Deck of cards

Flashlight/headlamp

Flushable wipes

Moist towelettes

Paper towels

Plastic zip-top bags

Sunglasses

Toilet paper

Water bottle

Wool blanket

OPTIONAL

Banjo

Barbecue grill

Binoculars

Field guides on bird, plant, and wildlife identification

Fishing rod and tackle

Lantern

Magnifying glass (for study-ing flowers, insects, etc.)

Maps (road, trail, topo-graphic, etc.)

APPENDIX B

Honorable Mention

Check out these nice campgrounds that didn't make the cut.

BRAZIL CREEK, Mark Twain National Forest Until recently Brazil Creek, while a bit neglected, was one of the nicest free campgrounds in Missouri. Featuring level grassy sites in a meadow next to its namesake creek, it was a pleasant place to hang out between hikes, mountain bike rides, or horseback excursions on the Berryman Trail. A few years ago the U.S. Forest Service pulled the tables, grills, and toilets from the camp, leaving only the lantern poles, and designated the site a trailhead. Camping is still allowed there, but you'll need to bring your own amenities to this pine-shaded camping spot.

HAZEL CREEK CAMPGROUND, Mark Twain National Forest Hazel Creek is not closed, but the U.S. Forest Service has allowed it to go to seed. The camp's toilets were removed, but tables, lantern poles, and fire grates are still in place. It's popular with equestrians and mountain bikers using the Ozark Trail, which runs right through the camp. There's no trash service, water, or toilets, but this campground nestled in a bend of Hazel Creek is a quiet, laid-back place off the beaten path.

CARVER, Buffalo National River This camp consists of eight walk-in sites in a partially shaded grassy expanse next to the Lower Buffalo River. There's a good swimming hole at Carver, and elk are often spotted in the open meadow to the east. It's not far from here to the climbing routes and scenic grandeur of Sam's Throne near Mt. Judea, or to the mountain bike and equestrian trails at Moccasin Gap. It's a little close to the highway, but it's not a busy road and there's hardly any traffic at all at night.

ERBIE CAMPGROUND, Buffalo National River Erbie is a victim of the budget sequester of 2013. It was closed in March of that year, but may have been reopened after our country's budget issues are resolved. Check the Buffalo National River website for updates. Located seven gravel-road miles from the nearest paved highway, Erbie is a nice off-the-beaten-path campground with group, walk-in, and park-in campsites. It's near good caving, excellent hiking, and several historic sites, and it offers canoe access to the Buffalo. For further information on activities near Erbie, see the profile on Ozark (page 136).

OZONE, Ozark National Forest There's not a lot to do at Ozone, but it's a wonderful place to spend a day or two. There are eight shady sites here, and each one is beautifully landscaped with stone-outlined tent pads and table sites. In the 1930s this was the site of the Civilian Conservation Corps Camp Ozone, where Company 1708 lived and worked in the surrounding forest. A fascinating self-guided interpretive trail explores the remains of the camp. It's mostly foundations scattered in the forest, but the goldfish pool in the shape of Arkansas

APPENDIX B

● ●

Honorable Mention *(continued)*

is interesting to see. The Ozark Highlands Trail runs right through camp, and at $3 per site Ozone is one of the best camping deals in the Ozarks. If you get tired of cooking, head a few miles south to the Ozone Burger Barn for good sandwiches and ice cream.

WOLF PEN, Ozark National Forest This small campground is another $3 wonder like Ozone. It's a bit more rustic—each site only has a lantern pole and fire ring—but if you need a table, you can wander over to Wolf Pen's five picnic sites. Wolf Pen is popular with river runners, but there's also great hiking nearby on the Ozark Highlands Trail and the Spy Rock Loop. Road biking on AR 123 is wonderful, and it's only a short jaunt up the road to Oark, where a charming general store offers great sandwiches, homemade pie, ice cream, and limited groceries. I recommend the buttermilk pie—it sounds terrible, but I was more than pleasantly surprised when I gave it a shot! For more information on the area, see the profile for Redding Recreation Area (page 156).

APPENDIX C

● ●

Sources of Information

BUFFALO NATIONAL RIVER
402 N. Walnut, Ste. 136
Harrison, AR 72601
870-365-2700
nps.gov/buff

**MARK TWAIN
NATIONAL FOREST**
401 Fairgrounds Rd.
Rolla, MO 65401
573-364-4621
www.fs.usda.gov/mtnf

**MISSOURI DEPARTMENT
OF CONSERVATION**
2901 W. Truman Blvd.
Jefferson City, MO 65109
573-751-4115
mdc.mo.gov

MISSOURI STATE PARKS
Department of Natural Resources
P.O. Box 176
Jefferson City, MO 65102
800-334-6946
mostateparks.com

**OZARK NATIONAL
SCENIC RIVERWAYS**
404 Watercress Dr.
P.O. Box 490
Van Buren, MO 63965
573-323-4236
nps.gov/ozar

**OZARK-ST. FRANCIS
NATIONAL FORESTS**
605 W. Main
Russellville, AR 72801
479-964-7200
www.fs.usda.gov/osfnf

OZARK TRAIL ASSOCIATION
406 W. High St.
Potosi, MO 63664
573-436-0540
ozarktrail.com

ST. CHARLES COUNTY PARKS
201 N. Second St., Ste. 510
St. Charles, MO 63301
636-949-7535
parks.sccmo.org/parks

APPENDIX D

● ●

Suggested Reading and Reference

Brent, Kelley, Jeff Bonney, and Cari Gerit. *Trails of Missouri State Parks.* Jefferson City, MO: Missouri Department of Natural Resources, 2012.

Carroll, Margo and Peggy Welch. *The Ozark Trail Guidebook.* 2nd ed. Crossville, TN: Enjoy The Journey, LLC, 2009.

Eddy, William B. and Richard O. Ballentine. *Hiking Kansas City: The Complete Guide to More Than 100 Hiking & Walking Trails in the Kansas City Area.* 5th ed. Rocheport, MO: Pebble Publishing, 2007.

Ernst, Tim. *Arkansas Hiking Trails: A Guide to 78 Selected Trails in "The Natural State."* 2nd ed. Pettigrew, AR: Cloudland Publishing, 1994.

Ernst, Tim. *Buffalo River Hiking Trails.* 3rd ed. Pettigrew, AR: Cloudland Publishing, 1998.

Ernst, Tim. *Ozark Highlands Trail Guide.* 5th ed. Pettigrew, AR: Cloudland Publishing, 2010.

Frey, Kelly and Steve Baron. *Trails of Missouri: A Guide to Hiking the Show-Me State.* St. Louis: Kelly Frey, 1995.

Gass, Ramon D. *Missouri Hiking Trails: A Detailed Guide to Selected Hiking Trails on Public Land in Missouri.* Jefferson City, MO: Missouri Department of Conservation, 1996.

Hawksley, Oz. *Missouri Ozark Waterways.* Jefferson City, MO: Missouri Department of Conservation, 1997.

Henry, Steve. *Mountain Bike! The Ozarks: A Guide to the Classic Trails.* 2nd ed. Birmingham, AL: Menasha Ridge Press, 2000.

Henry, Steve. *60 Hikes within 60 Miles: St. Louis.* Birmingham, AL: Menasha Ridge Press, 2011.

Kight, Teresa. *Conservation Trails: A Guide to Missouri Department of Conservation Hiking Trails.* Jefferson City, MO: Missouri Department of Conservation, 1999.

Lohraff, Kevin. *Hiking Missouri.* 2nd ed. Champaign, IL: Human Kinetics, 2009.

McPherson, Alan. *One Hundred Nature Walks in the Missouri Ozarks.* St. Louis: Cache River Press, 1997.

Molloy, Johnny. *50 Hikes in the Ozarks: Walks, Hikes, and Backpacks in the Mountains, Wilderness, and Geological Wonders of Arkansas and Missouri.* Woodstock, VT: Countryman Press, 2008.

Schirle, John. *Best Tent Camping: Illinois.* Birmingham, AL: Menasha Ridge Press, 2009.

INDEX

● ●

DEAR CUSTOMERS AND FRIENDS,

SUPPORTING YOUR INTEREST IN OUTDOOR ADVENTURE, travel, and an active lifestyle is central to our operations, from the authors we choose to the locations we detail to the way we design our books. Menasha Ridge Press was incorporated in 1982 by a group of veteran outdoorsmen and professional outfitters. For many years now, we've specialized in creating books that benefit the outdoors enthusiast.

Almost immediately, Menasha Ridge Press earned a reputation for revolutionizing outdoors- and travel-guidebook publishing. For such activities as canoeing, kayaking, hiking, backpacking, and mountain biking, we established new standards of quality that transformed the whole genre, resulting in outdoor-recreation guides of great sophistication and solid content. Menasha Ridge continues to be outdoor publishing's greatest innovator.

The folks at Menasha Ridge Press are as at home on a white-water river or mountain trail as they are editing a manuscript. The books we build for you are the best they can be, because we're responding to your needs. Plus, we use and depend on them ourselves.

We look forward to seeing you on the river or the trail. If you'd like to contact us directly, join in at www.trekalong.com or visit us at www.menasharidge.com. We thank you for your interest in our books and the natural world around us all.

SAFE TRAVELS,

Bob Sehlinger

BOB SEHLINGER
PUBLISHER

ABOUT THE AUTHOR

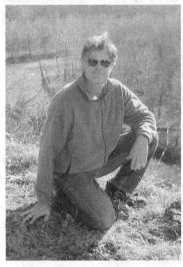

Steve Henry grew up on a farm in the roll-ing hills of central Kansas, spending much of his youth working under the blue skies of the plains. After earning bachelor's degrees in marketing and agricul-tural economics at Kansas State University, he served a sentence of seven years in the offices of an insurance company. Missing the outdoor life, he finally left the insurance company in 1985 to cycle across the conti-nent twice, including one trek from Anchorage, Alaska, to Key West, Florida. Since then he has organized triathlons, led bicycle and backpack tours, written freelance outdoor articles, and enjoyed many camp-ing trips. If you spot a tall, middle-aged guy playing the banjo badly in a campsite near yours, it could be Steve. Wander on over for a visit, and ask him to put away the banjo if you think he's threatening the camp's five-star rating for quiet. Steve is also the author of *60 Hikes within 60 Miles: St. Louis* (Menasha Ridge Press). When not explor-ing the Ozarks, Steve admires the countryside from a Peterbilt 379. You can contact him at **stevehenryoutdoors@yahoo.com** or at his website, **stevehenryoutdoors.com.**

Printed in the USA
CPSIA information can be obtained
at www.ICGtesting.com
JSHW060755140424
61126JS00006B/14